T0362284

ORTHOPEDIC CLINICS OF NORTH AMERICA

www.orthopedic.theclinics.com

Managing Comorbidities

July 2023 • Volume 54 • Number 3

ELSEVIER

1600 John F. Kennedy Boulevard • Suite 1800 • Philadelphia, Pennsylvania, 19103-2899.

http://www.orthopedic.theclinics.com

ORTHOPEDIC CLINICS OF NORTH AMERICA Volume 54, Number 3
July 2023 ISSN 0030-5898, ISBN-13: 978-0-323-93897-6

Editor: Megan Ashdown
Developmental Editor: Shivank Joshi

Orthopedic Clinics of North America (ISSN 0030-5898) is published quarterly by Elsevier Inc., 360 Park Avenue South, New York, NY 10010-1710. Months of issue are January, April, July, and October. Business and Editorial Offices: 1600 John F. Kennedy Blvd., Suite 1800, Philadelphia, PA 19103-2899. Customer Service Office: 3251 Riverport Lane, Maryland Heights, MO 63043. Periodicals postage paid at New York, NY and additional mailing offices. Subscription prices are $365.00 per year for (US individuals), $834.00 per year for (US institutions), $433.00 per year (Canadian individuals), $1,019.00 per year (Canadian institutions), $501.00 per year (international individuals), $1,019.00 per year (international institutions), $100.00 per year (US students), $100.00 per year for (Canadian students), $220.00 per year for (international students). Foreign air speed delivery is included in all *Clinics* subscription prices. All prices are subject to change without notice. **POSTMASTER:** Send change of address to *Orthopedic Clinics of North America*, **Elsevier Health Sciences Division, Subscription Customer Service, 3251 Riverport Lane, Maryland Heights, MO 63043. Customer Service (orders, claims, online, change of address): Elsevier Health Sciences Division, Subscription Customer Service, 3251 Riverport Lane, Maryland Heights, MO 63043. Tel: 1-800-654-2452 (U.S. and Canada); 314-447-8871 (outside U.S. and Canada). Fax: 314-447-8029. E-mail:** journalscustomerservice-usa@elsevier.com **(for print support);** journalsonlinesupport-usa@elsevier.com **(for online support).**

Reprints. For copies of 100 or more, of articles in this publication, please contact the Commercial Reprints Department, Elsevier Inc., 360 Park Avenue South, New York, NY 10010-1710. Tel.: 212-633-3874; Fax: 212-633-3820; E-mail: reprints@elsevier.com.

Orthopedic Clinics of North America is covered in *MEDLINE/PubMed (Index Medicus), Cinahl, Excerpta Medica, and Cumulative Index to Nursing and Allied Health Literature.*

EDITORIAL BOARD

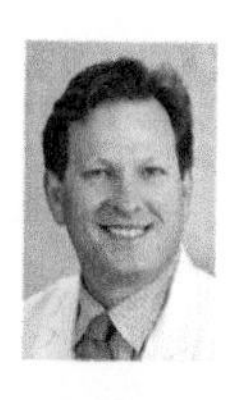

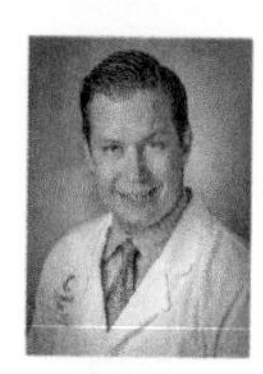

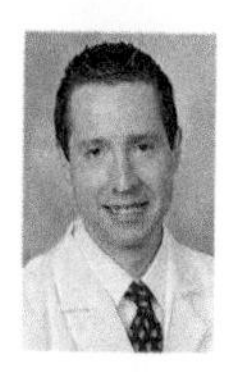

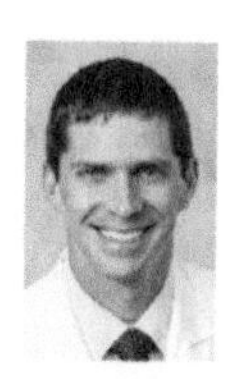

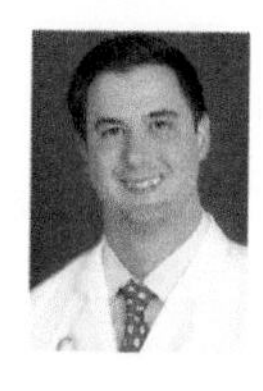

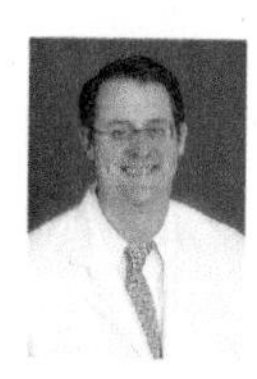

CONTRIBUTORS

EDITOR

FREDRICK M. AZAR, MD
Editor-in-Chief, Orthopedic Clinics of North America, Campbell Clinic Department of Orthopaedic Surgery and Biomedical Engineering, University of Tennessee Health Science Center, Memphis, Tennessee

AUTHORS

BENJAMIN J. AVERKAMP, MD
Ortho Carolina Hip and Knee Center, Atrium Health - Musculoskeletal Institute, Charlotte, North Carolina

CHARLES LOWRY BARNES, MD
Department of Orthopaedic Surgery, University of Arkansas for Medical Sciences, Little Rock, Arkansas

MARIA F. BOZOGHLIAN, MD
Research Associate, Department of Orthopedics and Rehabilitation, University of Iowa, Iowa City, Iowa

LAUREN BURGE, MD
Assistant Professor of Pediatrics, Division of Child Abuse, The University of Tennessee Health Science Center, Memphis, Tennessee

JAMES H. CALANDRUCCIO, MD
Campbell Clinic Department of Orthopaedic Surgery and Biomedical Engineering, The University of Tennessee Health Science Center, Memphis, Tennessee

ANNETTE CARLISLE, MD
Assistant Professor of Pediatrics, Division of Allergy and Immunology, The University of Tennessee Health Science Center, Memphis, Tennessee

MARIA CARRILLO-MARQUEZ, MD
Associate Professor of Pediatrics, Division of Infectious Diseases, The University of Tennessee Health Science Center, Memphis, Tennessee

JESSICA L. CHURCHILL, MD
Department of Orthopedic Surgery, Cleveland Clinic Foundation, Cleveland, Ohio

MATTHEW R. COLATRUGLIO, MD
Department of Orthopedic Surgery, Campbell Clinic, The University of Tennessee Health Science Center, Memphis, Tennessee; Campbell Clinic Orthopedics, Germantown, Tennessee

SAM DAGOGO-JACK, MD, DSc
Professor of Medicine and Chief, Division of Endocrinology, Diabetes and Metabolism, The University of Tennessee Health Science Center, Memphis, Tennessee

ZACHARY R. DILTZ, MD
Department of Orthopedic Surgery, Campbell Clinic, The University of Tennessee Health Science Center, Memphis, Tennessee; Campbell Clinic Orthopedics, Germantown, Tennessee

VAHID ENTEZARI, MD
Assistant Professor of Surgery, Cleveland Clinic Lerner College of Medicine, Case Western Reserve University School of Medicine, Department of Orthopedic Surgery, Cleveland Clinic Foundation, Cleveland, Ohio

ANDREW FRAVAL, MD, FRACS
Rothman Institute, Thomas Jefferson University, Philadelphia, Pennsylvania

JASON C. HO, MD
Assistant Professor of Surgery, Cleveland Clinic Lerner College of Medicine, Case Western Reserve University School of Medicine, Department of Orthopedic Surgery, Cleveland Clinic Foundation, Cleveland, Ohio

HAYDEN S. HOLBROOK, MD
Campbell Clinic Department of Orthopaedic Surgery and Biomedical Engineering, The University of Tennessee Health Science Center, Memphis, Tennessee

WILLIAM J. HOZACK, MD
Rothman Institute Orthopaedics at Thomas Jefferson University Hospital, Philadelphia, Pennsylvania

DEIRDRE JAMES, MD
Assistant Professor of Medicine, Division of Endocrinology, Diabetes and Metabolism, The University of Tennessee Health Science Center, Memphis, Tennessee

JOSEF E. JOLISSAINT, MD
Ortho Carolina Hip and Knee Center, Atrium Health - Musculoskeletal Institute, Charlotte, North Carolina

MARIA S. KAMMIRE, MD
Ortho Carolina Hip and Knee Center, Atrium Health - Musculoskeletal Institute, Charlotte, North Carolina

DILASHA KATWAL, MD
Clinical Endocrinology Fellow, Division of Endocrinology, Diabetes and Metabolism, The University of Tennessee Health Science Center, Memphis, Tennessee

MATEO J. KIRWAN, MD
Department of Orthopedic Surgery, Campbell Clinic, The University of Tennessee Health Science Center, Memphis, Tennessee; Campbell Clinic Orthopedics, Germantown, Tennessee

ELLIOT N. KONRADE, MD
Department of Orthopedic Surgery, Campbell Clinic, The University of Tennessee Health Science Center, Memphis, Tennessee; Campbell Clinic Orthopedics, Germantown, Tennessee

RYAN LEDUC, MD
Loyola University Medical Center, Maywood, Illinois

PATRICK COLE McGREGOR, MD
Loyola University Medical Center, Maywood, Illinois

SIMON C. MEARS, MD, PhD
Department of Orthopaedic Surgery, University of Arkansas for Medical Sciences, Little Rock, Arkansas

GRACE B. NELSON, MD
Assistant Professor, Pediatrics, The University of Tennessee Health Science Center, Memphis, Tennessee

CONNER J. PAEZ, MD
Department of Orthopedic Surgery, Cleveland Clinic Foundation, Cleveland, Ohio

JAVAD PARVIZI, MD, FRCS
Rothman Orthopaedic Institute, Thomas Jefferson University Hospital, Philadelphia, Pennsylvania

BRENDAN M. PATTERSON, MD, MPH
Associate Professor, Department of Orthopedics and Rehabilitation, University of Iowa, Iowa City, Iowa

ERIC T. RICCHETTI, MD
Associate Professor of Surgery, Cleveland Clinic Lerner College of Medicine, Case Western Reserve University School of Medicine, Department of Orthopedic Surgery, Cleveland Clinic Foundation, Cleveland, Ohio

NATHANIEL G. ROGERS, MD
Assistant Professor of Internal Medicine and Pediatrics, Division of Pediatric Hospital Medicine, The University of Tennessee Health Science Center, Memphis, Tennessee

CATHERINE D. SANDERS, MD
Assistant Professor of Pediatrics, Division of Pulmonology, The University of Tennessee Health Science Center, Memphis, Tennessee

AARON SESLER, BS
Department of Orthopaedic Surgery, University of Arkansas for Medical Sciences, Little Rock, Arkansas

BRYAN D. SPRINGER, MD
Attending Orthopaedic Surgeon, Ortho Carolina Hip and Knee Center, Atrium Health - Musculoskeletal Institute, Charlotte, North Carolina

JEFFREY B. STAMBOUGH, MD
Department of Orthopaedic Surgery, University of Arkansas for Medical Sciences, Little Rock, Arkansas

BENJAMIN M. STRONACH, MS, MD
Department of Orthopaedic Surgery, University of Arkansas for Medical Sciences, Little Rock, Arkansas

KATHRYN M. SUMPTER, MD
Associate Professor, Pediatrics, The University of Tennessee Health Science Center, Memphis, Tennessee

SAAD TARABICHI, MD
Rothman Orthopaedic Institute, Thomas Jefferson University Hospital, Philadelphia, Pennsylvania

KIRK M. THOMPSON, MD
Department of Orthopedic Surgery, Campbell Clinic, The University of Tennessee Health Science Center, Memphis, Tennessee; Campbell Clinic Orthopedics, Germantown, Tennessee

ERIC J. WEST, MD
Department of Orthopedic Surgery, Campbell Clinic, The University of Tennessee Health Science Center, Memphis, Tennessee; Campbell Clinic Orthopedics, Germantown, Tennessee

CONTENTS

MANAGING COMORBIDITIES

FORTHCOMING ISSUES

October 2023
Perioperative Pain Management
Michael J. Beebe, Clayton C. Bettin, Tyler J. Brolin, James H. Calandruccio, Christopher T. Cosgrove, Benjamin J. Grear, Benjamin M. Mauck, William M. Mihalko, Benjamin Sheffer, Kirk M. Thompson, and Marcus Ford, *Editors*

January 2024
Intraoperative Challenges
Michael J. Beebe, Clayton C. Bettin, Tyler J. Brolin, James H. Calandruccio, Christopher T. Cosgrove, Benjamin J. Grear, Benjamin M. Mauck, William M. Mihalko, Benjamin Sheffer, Kirk M. Thompson, Marcus Ford, and William J. Weller, *Editors*

April 2024
Infections
Michael J. Beebe, Clayton C. Bettin, Tyler J. Brolin, James H. Calandruccio, Christopher T. Cosgrove, Benjamin J. Grear, Benjamin M. Mauck, William M. Mihalko, Benjamin Sheffer, Kirk M.Thompson, Marcus Ford, and William J. Weller, *Editors*

RECENT ISSUES

April 2023
Technological Advances
Michael J. Beebe, Clayton C. Bettin, Tyler J. Brolin, James H. Calandruccio, Christopher T. Cosgrove, Benjamin J. Grear, Benjamin M. Mauck, William M. Mihalko, Benjamin Sheffer, Kirk M. Thompson, and Marcus Ford, *Editors*

January 2023
Tumors
Michael J. Beebe, Clayton C. Bettin, Tyler J. Brolin, James H. Calandruccio, Christopher T. Cosgrove, Benjamin J. Grear, Benjamin M. Mauck, William M. Mihalko, Benjamin Sheffer, Kirk M. Thompson, and Patrick C. Toy, *Editors*

October 2022
Musculoskeletal Disorders
Michael J. Beebe, Clayton C. Bettin, Tyler J. Brolin, James H. Calandruccio, Christopher T. Cosgrove, Benjamin J. Grear, Benjamin M. Mauck, William M. Mihalko, Benjamin Sheffer, Kirk M. Thompson, and Patrick C. Toy, *Editors*

Erratum

In the April 2023 *Orthopedic Clinics* (Volume 54, number 2) article, "Intraoperative Navigation and Robotics in Pediatric Spinal Deformity," pages 201-207, an author's middle initial was mistakenly transposed. The author should be listed as "Benjamin W. Sheffer."

Orthop Clin N Am 54 (2023) xv
https://doi.org/10.1016/j.ocl.2023.03.001

PREFACE

Managing Comorbidities

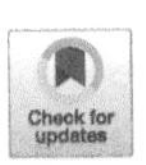

As we all know, comorbidities can complicate the treatment and management of orthopedic problems. These unrelated medical conditions also can lead to surgical complications, affect recuperation time, and even increase the risk of death. This issue examines the effect of some major comorbidities—including obesity, diabetes, gout, and peripheral vascular disease (PVD)—on elderly, pediatric, and rural orthopedic patients and explores how to best deal with them to achieve optimal outcomes.

Diabetes is one of the world's fastest-growing diseases, afflicting over 37 million Americans and leading to more than 100,000 lower-extremity amputations annually in the United States. Katwal and colleagues discuss how optimization of glycemic control and comorbid risk factors can help lessen the early foot lesions, peripheral neuropathy, and PVD that frequently lead to such amputations. McGregor and LeDuc, meanwhile, explore the proper management and multidisciplinary approach that should be taken before diabetic patients undergo elective foot-and-ankle surgery.

Treatment regiments for patients with type 1 diabetes (T1D) have become more complex, with newer insulin analogues and technology becoming increasingly effective at maintaining glucose in target range. Nelson and Sumpter believe that T1D technology should be used more widely during hospitalization and surgery to ameliorate the stress responses that can lead to glucose variability. Children, who are the main T1D patients, can have complicated orthopedic issues. Sanders and Burge explain how early consultation and collaboration with pediatric subspecialists will expedite a young patient's care.

At the other end of the age spectrum, bone fractures are common problems that can lead to functional decline. Tarabichi and Parvizi discuss the multidisciplinary approach that is needed to manage geriatric patients, who are prone to bone-breaking falls.

Gout, the most common form of inflammatory arthritis, can be alleviated by lifestyle changes and urate-lowering therapy. Holbrook and Calandruccio focus on how to treat common signs of gout in the upper extremity.

Morbid obesity puts hip and knee arthroplasty candidates at great risk of surgical complications and poorer outcomes, so some surgeons set a strict body mass index cutoff of 40 for patients. Jolissaint and colleagues argue, however, that such cutoffs might not be justified or ethical. Different challenges exist for rural residents who need total joint arthroplasty—optimization for surgery can be more difficult because of lack of access to proper surgical institution and household income. Sesler and colleagues advocate policy initiatives that will reduce socioeconomic differences in rural areas and note that remote technologies can help with medical access.

PVD can complicate wound healing and increase infections after total knee arthroplasty. Fraval and Hozack review the pathophysiology of PVD and current management strategies and provide diagnostic pearls. Complications also can ensue after spinal surgery if comorbidities aren't managed properly. Diltz and colleagues write that obesity, older age, substance use, mood disorders, and a host of other medical challenges need to be appropriately dealt with so that optimal clinical outcomes are obtained.

The shoulder-and-elbow section looks at the importance of preoperative management of comorbidities before total shoulder arthroplasty, which has become more common as people live

Orthop Clin N Am 54 (2023) xvii–xviii
https://doi.org/10.1016/j.ocl.2023.05.001
0030-5898/23/© 2023 Published by Elsevier Inc.

longer and stay active. Churchill and colleagues point out that identifying modifiable medical conditions, such as cardiovascular issues and anemia, before surgery might decrease costs and improve the overall outcome. Patterson and Bozoghlian, meanwhile, examine the risk factors associated with recurrent rotator cuff tears, with which surgeons should be familiar.

We thank the authors for their valuable information and hope that readers will find these topics helpful in their practices.

Frederick M. Azar, MD
Campbell Clinic
Department of Orthopaedic Surgery and Biomedical Engineering
University of Tennessee Health Science Center
1211 Union Avenue, Suite 510
Memphis, TN 38104, USA

E-mail address:
fazar@campbellclinic.com

Knee and Hip Reconstruction

Preventing the Impact of Hyperglycemia and Diabetes on Patients Undergoing Total Joint Arthroplasty

Saad Tarabichi, MD, Javad Parvizi, MD, FRCS*

KEYWORDS

• Diabetes mellitus • Hyperglycemia • Total joint arthroplasty • Periprosthetic joint infection

KEY POINTS

- Diabetes mellitus continues to compromise the success of total joint arthroplasty.
- A growing number of presumed "nondiabetic" patients develop hyperglycemia perioperatively.
- HbA1c% may not be as relaible as previously believed in identifying patients with poor glycemic control.

INTRODUCTION

Diabetes mellitus is a common medical ailment that affects the well-being of roughly 9.3% of the adult population worldwide.[1] In the United States alone, the number of patients with diabetes is expected to double over the next 20 years, reaching an all-time high of approximately 44 million.[2] Concurrently, primary and revision total joint arthroplasty (TJA) are increasingly popular procedures and account for a substantial portion of annual medicare spending.[3,4]

Preoperative optimization of modifiable host factors in patients undergoing elective orthopedic procedures has become standard-of-care.[5] In particular, diabetes mellitus is a common comorbid condition in this patient population and has been shown to increase the risk of complications such as periprosthetic joint infection (PJI) and death.[6] Furthermore, a recent study demonstrated that greater than 30% of patients undergoing TJA had previously undiagnosed hyperglycemia.[7]

In an effort to mitigate the impact of poor glycemic control on patients undergoing TJA, recent clinical practice guidelines have helped standardize our management of patients considered high risk in this setting.[8] Notwithstanding, as the number of TJA procedures performed annually continues to rise, so will the rate of complications secondary to medical comorbidities, especially diabetes mellitus.[9,10]

This article will serve as an overview of current practices and protocols employed to help prevent the impact of hyperglycemia and diabetes on the outcomes of patients undergoing TJA.

PATIENT EVALUATION OVERVIEW

It is well-established that a large number of patients undergoing TJA have poor glycemic control.[7] Although it was previously believed that only diabetic patients were at an increased risk of postoperative hyperglycemia, a growing body of evidence has suggested that up to 40% of all patients undergoing TJA develop hyperglycemia perioperatively.[11] In addition to this, several patient-specific factors have been shown to be predictors of substantial increases in blood glucose levels following TJA. These include but are not limited to revision TJA, obesity, and male sex.[12] Of note, recent studies have demonstrated that higher glucose variability increased the risk for complications in patients undergoing primary and revision TJA.[13,14]

Rothman Orthopaedic Institute at Thomas Jefferson University Hospital, Philadelphia, PA, USA
* Corresponding author. 125 South 9th Street, Suite 1000, Philadelphia, PA 19107.
E-mail address: javadparvizi@gmail.com

Orthop Clin N Am 54 (2023) 247–250
https://doi.org/10.1016/j.ocl.2023.02.008

Currently, HbA1c% is the gold standard for determining glycemic control in diabetic patients undergoing surgery.[15] In a recent study, a HbA1c % cutoff of 7.7% was found to be the most predictive of PJI development at 1 year following TJA.[16] However, a growing body of evidence has shown that HbA1c% may not be as reliable as previously believed in identifying patients with poor glycemic control.[17] Similarly, several studies in the literature have failed to identify a correlation between HbA1c% levels and acute PJI rates (within 90 days).[18] Furthermore, HbA1c% levels can take up to 3 months to respond to treatment and thus lack the sensitivity necessary to appropriately determine the degree of glycemic control in patients undergoing TJA.[19] More recently, there have been data to suggest that fructosamine, a glucose byproduct, may be more suitable for identifying poor glycemic control in this patient population.[20] In one study, a fructosamine reading of ≥293 μmol/L in patients undergoing TJA was an independent risk factor for surgical site infection, reoperation, and readmission.[17]

PREVENTIVE TECHNIQUES

Preoperative

In addition to conventional health promotion techniques, carbohydrate restriction in the weeks leading up to surgery is a well-recognized method of hyperglycemia prevention.[21] In a recent study, the authors demonstrated that 2 weeks of carbohydrate restriction in diabetic patients resulted in a significant reduction in fasting HbA1c and fasting blood glucose levels on the day of surgery.[22] In addition to this, a separate study found that primary TJA patients who were prescribed carbohydrate-restricted diets had significantly lower blood glucose readings throughout the period of their admission.[23] Moreover, there have been data to suggest that giving nondiabetic patients carbohydrate-restricted diets, before and during their admission, can significantly reduce the rate of postoperative hyperglycemia (18% vs 23%, $P < .01$).[24]

Perioperative

In recent years, we have identified several modifiable factors that have been shown to increase the risk of hyperglycemia perioperatively. In one study, the authors demonstrated that the number of glucocorticoid doses given intraoperatively correlated directly with higher postoperative blood glucose readings.[25,26] In addition to this, there has been evidence to suggest that patients administered general anesthesia experience more frequent blood glucose fluctuations and are more likely to develop hyperglycemia when compared with patients managed with spinal anesthesia.[27] Furthermore, in contrast to conventional anesthetic agents, non-barbiturate hypnotics and benzodiazepines have been shown to produce significant reductions in postoperative glucose readings.[28]

Intraoperative

Blood glucose monitoring at regular intervals throughout the duration of any surgical procedure has become standard-of-care.[29] Although most clinical practice guidelines allow for some degree of hyperglycemia intraoperatively, there is a growing body of evidence to support the administration of insulin in patients with a blood glucose reading of greater than 150 mg/dL.[30] Similarly, a recent study found that patients who had their blood glucose levels maintained to less than 150 mg/dL for the entirety of their procedure experienced significantly lower rates of infection postoperatively.[31]

NEW DEVELOPMENTS

Glycated albumin (GA) has garnered interest in recent years as a marker of glycemic control in patients undergoing surgery.[32] Given its relatively short half-life, GA has been shown to be more sensitive than traditional HbA1c in identifying glycemic control.[33] Furthermore, unlike fructosamine and HbA1c, the measurement of GA is more standardized and has not been shown to be influenced by the concentrations of other serum proteins.[34,35] Although the utility of GA has only been demonstrated in the management of patients with diabetes, its superior accuracy has resulted in its widespread incorporation across endocrinology.[36] Currently, our institution, in collaboration with other institutions, is conducting a multicenter prospective study to determine the prognostic utility of GA in patients undergoing primary TJA.[37]

SUMMARY

Diabetes and hyperglycemia continue to compromise the success of surgical procedures worldwide. Furthermore, as the annual volume of TJA procedures continues to expand, the rate of complications secondary to poor glycemic control is also expected to rise. Therefore, it is paramount for orthopedic surgeons to continue to familiarize themselves with the best available evidence in an effort to prevent the impact of this disease process on patients undergoing primary and revision TJA.

CLINICS CARE POINTS

- Hyperglycemia and diabetes in patients undergoing TJA is increasingly common.
- Poor glycemic control is a well-recognized risk factor for several complications, including death.
- We have identified several factors that can be modified to help mitigate the impact of this disease process on the outcomes of patients undergoing TJA.
- Orthopedic surgeons must remain up to date on the best available evidence in this setting.

DISCLOSURE

No relevant disclosures.

REFERENCES

1. Saeedi P, Petersohn I, Salpea P, et al. Global and regional diabetes prevalence estimates for 2019 and projections for 2030 and 2045: Results from the International Diabetes Federation Diabetes Atlas, 9th edition. Diabetes Res Clin Pract 2019; 157:107843.
2. National Diabetes Statistics Report 2020. Estimates of diabetes and its burden in the United States. Published online 2020.
3. Kurtz S. Prevalence of primary and revision total hip and knee arthroplasty in the United States from 1990 through 2002. J Bone Joint Surg 2005;87(7): 1487.
4. Kurtz S, Ong K, Lau E, et al. Projections of primary and revision hip and knee arthroplasty in the United States from 2005 to 2030. J Bone Joint Surg Am 2007;89(4):780–5.
5. Bernstein DN, Liu TC, Winegar AL, et al. Evaluation of a preoperative optimization protocol for primary hip and knee arthroplasty patients. J Arthroplasty 2018;33(12):3642–8.
6. Bolognesi MP, Marchant MH, Viens NA, et al. The impact of diabetes on perioperative patient outcomes after total hip and total knee arthroplasty in the United States. J Arthroplasty 2008; 23(6):92–8.
7. Shohat N, Goswami K, Tarabichi M, et al. All patients should be screened for diabetes before total joint arthroplasty. J Arthroplasty 2018;33(7):2057–61.
8. Lamanna DL, McDonnell ME, Chen AF, et al. Perioperative identification and management of hyperglycemia in orthopaedic surgery. JBJS 2022; 104(23):2117.
9. Kurtz SM, Ong KL, Lau E, et al. Prosthetic joint infection risk after TKA in the Medicare population. Clin Orthop Relat Res 2010;468(1):52–6.
10. Kurtz SM, Lau E, Watson H, et al. Economic burden of periprosthetic joint infection in the United States. J Arthroplasty 2012;27(8 Suppl):61–5.e1.
11. Jämsen E, Nevalainen PI, Eskelinen A, et al. Risk factors for perioperative hyperglycemia in primary hip and knee replacements. Acta Orthop 2015; 86(2):175–82.
12. Gallagher JM, Erich RA, Gattermeyer R, et al. Postoperative hyperglycemia can be safely and effectively controlled in both diabetic and nondiabetic patients with use of a subcutaneous insulin protocol. JB JS Open Access 2017;2(1):e0008.
13. Shohat N, Foltz C, Restrepo C, et al. Increased postoperative glucose variability is associated with adverse outcomes following orthopaedic surgery. Bone Joint Lett J 2018;100-B(8):1125–32.
14. Goh GS, Shohat N, Abdelaal MS, et al. Serum glucose variability increases the risk of complications following aseptic revision hip and knee arthroplasty. J Bone Joint Surg Am 2022;104(18):1614–20.
15. American Diabetes Association. 6. Glycemic targets. Diabetes Care 2014;38(Supplement_1):S33–40.
16. Tarabichi M, Shohat N, Kheir MM, et al. Determining the threshold for hba1c as a predictor for adverse outcomes after total joint arthroplasty: a multicenter, retrospective study. J Arthroplasty 2017;32(9S):263–7.e1.
17. Shohat N, Tarabichi M, Tan TL, et al. John insall award: fructosamine is a better glycaemic marker compared with glycated haemoglobin (HBA1C) in predicting adverse outcomes following total knee arthroplasty: a prospective multicentre study. Bone Joint Lett J 2019;101-B(7_Supple_C):3–9.
18. Capozzi JD, Lepkowsky ER, Callari MM, et al. The prevalence of diabetes mellitus and routine hemoglobin a1c screening in elective total joint arthroplasty patients. J Arthroplasty 2017;32(1):304–8.
19. Sherwani SI, Khan HA, Ekhzaimy A, et al. Significance of HbA1c Test in diagnosis and prognosis of diabetic patients. Biomark Insights 2016;11:95–104.
20. Shohat N, Goswami K, Breckenridge L, et al. Fructosamine is a valuable marker for glycemic control and predicting adverse outcomes following total hip arthroplasty: a prospective multi-institutional investigation. Sci Rep 2021;11(1):2227.
21. Feinman RD, Pogozelski WK, Astrup A, et al. Dietary carbohydrate restriction as the first approach in diabetes management: critical review and evidence base. Nutrition 2015;31(1):1–13.
22. Boden G, Sargrad K, Homko C, et al. Effect of a low-carbohydrate diet on appetite, blood glucose levels, and insulin resistance in obese patients with type 2 diabetes. Ann Intern Med 2005;142(6): 403–11.

23. Ferrera HK, Jones TE, Schudrowitz NJ, et al. Perioperative dietary restriction of carbohydrates in the management of blood glucose levels in patients undergoing total knee replacement. J Arthroplasty 2019;34(6):1105–9.
24. Chen AF, Schwab. Consistent carbohydrate diet normalizes blood glucose levels in non-diabetics after orthopaedic surgery. Presented at the 19th European Society of Sports Traumatology, Knee Surgery and Arthroscopy (ESSKA). Published online May 15, 2021.
25. Clore JN, Thurby-Hay L. Glucocorticoid-induced hyperglycemia. Endocr Pract 2009;15(5):469–74.
26. Varady NH, Schwab PE, Jones T, et al. Optimal timing of glucose measurements after total joint arthroplasty. J Arthroplasty 2019;34(7S):S152–8.
27. Rehman HU, Mohammed K. Perioperative management of diabetic patients. Curr Surg 2003;60(6):607–11.
28. Palermo NE, Gianchandani RY, McDonnell ME, et al. Stress hyperglycemia during surgery and anesthesia: pathogenesis and clinical implications. Curr Diab Rep 2016;16(3):33.
29. Raju TA, Torjman MC, Goldberg ME. Perioperative blood glucose monitoring in the general surgical population. J Diabetes Sci Technol 2009;3(6):1282–7.
30. Duggan EW, Carlson K, Umpierrez GE. Perioperative hyperglycemia management: an update. Anesthesiology 2017;126(3):547–60.
31. de Vries FEE, Gans SL, Solomkin JS, et al. Meta-analysis of lower perioperative blood glucose target levels for reduction of surgical-site infection. Br J Surg 2017;104(2):e95–105.
32. Selvin E, Francis LMA, Ballantyne CM, et al. Nontraditional markers of glycemia: associations with microvascular conditions. Diabetes Care 2011;34(4):960–7.
33. Hashimoto K, Osugi T, Noguchi S, et al. A1C but not serum glycated albumin is elevated because of iron deficiency in late pregnancy in diabetic women. Diabetes Care 2010;33(3):509–11.
34. Danese E, Montagnana M, Nouvenne A, et al. Advantages and pitfalls of fructosamine and glycated albumin in the diagnosis and treatment of diabetes. J Diabetes Sci Technol 2015;9(2):169–76.
35. Montagnana M, Paleari R, Danese E, et al. Evaluation of biological variation of glycated albumin (GA) and fructosamine in healthy subjects. Clin Chim Acta 2013;423:1–4.
36. Desouza CV, Holcomb RG, Rosenstock J, et al. Results of a study comparing glycated albumin to other glycemic indices. The Journal of Clinical Endocrinology & Metabolism 2020;105(3):677–87.
37. FARE Finalists Announced | AAHKS. 2021. Available at: https://www.aahks.org/fare-finalists-announced/. Accessed January 14, 2023.

An Update on the Management and Optimization of the Patient with Morbid Obesity Undergoing Hip or Knee Arthroplasty

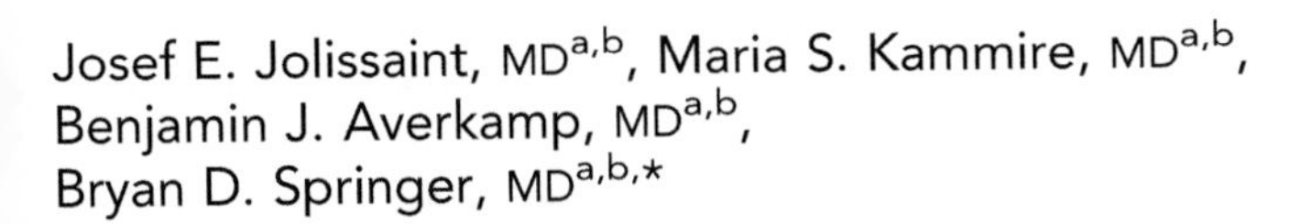

Josef E. Jolissaint, MD[a,b], Maria S. Kammire, MD[a,b],
Benjamin J. Averkamp, MD[a,b],
Bryan D. Springer, MD[a,b,*]

KEYWORDS

• Obesity • BMI • Joint replacement surgery • Arthroplasty • Bariatric surgery

KEY POINTS

- The prevalence of obesity is increasing at an alarming rate, and the prevalence of obesity is even higher in an arthroplasty population.
- Historically, a BMI > 40 has been linked to an increased risk of complications related to both primary and revision hip and knee arthroplasty.
- Recently, there have been concerns regarding limiting access to care for obese patients and difficulty losing weight with osteoarthritis.
- The literature surrounding the benefits and risks of bariatric surgery is not conclusive.
- We recommend a balanced approach emphasizing the medical optimization of all patients as opposed to a strict cutoff for surgery.

INTRODUCTION

According to the 2017 to 2020 National Health and Nutrition Examination Survey (NHANES), the prevalence of obesity in the United States is at a record high of 42%.[1] Although alarming, this statistic is not entirely unexpected given the country's gradual rise in obesity over the past several decades. In 1999, the Centers for Disease Control and Prevention recognized the obesity epidemic as a national problem, spurring the first generation of interventions for obesity prevention and control.[2] Despite billions of dollars in funding, legislative changes, and public health initiatives, the trajectory of American obesity has not waivered. Between 1999 and 2020, the prevalence of obesity (body mass index [BMI] 30) in the United States increased from 30.5% to 41.9%, with severe obesity (BMI 40) increasing from 4.7% to 9.2%.[1] Predictions show that by 2030, nearly 1 in 2 adults in this country will qualify as obese.[3]

Obesity has been linked to a broad spectrum of medical conditions, most of which stem from the systemic effects of adipose tissue on the body. Adipose cells release numerous types of

Disclosure
The authors have nothing to disclose.

[a] Ortho Carolina Hip and Knee Center, Charlotte, NC, USA; [b] Atrium Health - Musculoskeletal Institute, Charlotte, NC, USA
* Corresponding author.
E-mail address: bryan.springer@orthocarolina.com

Orthop Clin N Am 54 (2023) 251–257
https://doi.org/10.1016/j.ocl.2023.02.010
0030-5898/23/

proinflammatory cytokines and adipokines, which over time create a state of chronic, low-grade inflammation.[4] This baseline metabolic inflammation has been linked to many comorbidities, including diabetes, cardiovascular disease, hypertension, asthma, and arthritis. The disruption in physiologic growth factor and hormone levels associated with obesity has also been linked to at least 13 different types of cancer.[5] Obesity is now one of the leading causes of preventable cancers and preventable deaths, second only to smoking, and is poised to overtake it as the primary cause in the next 20 years.[6–8]

Alongside obesity-related comorbidities, obesity is also strongly associated with the development of osteoarthritis (OA). In combination with an increased mechanical load on joints, the aforementioned adipokines and proinflammatory cytokines can lead to destruction of cartilage and arthritic changes. In a study of almost 2 million subjects, being overweight or obese increased the risk of OA of the hip and knee, with a BMI of 35 increasing knee OA by almost 5-fold.[9] In fact, the prevalence of obesity in patients requiring total knee arthroplasty (TKA) was found to be greater than that of the general population and was found to be steadily increasing between 2000 and 2008.[10] This growing population of young, obese, and sick patients presents a unique dilemma for orthopedic surgeons performing joint replacement, as obesity levels as well as the demand for joint replacement are only expected to rise further.[11]

COMPLICATIONS IN TOTAL JOINT ARTHROPLASTY IN OBESE PATIENTS

As the prevalence of obesity has continued to rise throughout the last 40 years, concern has grown regarding the increased risk of performing arthroplasty in this population. A plethora of literature has been published in the last 10 years demonstrating increased rates of complications and worse outcomes in obese patients undergoing primary and revision joint-replacement surgeries. Malinzak and colleagues evaluated 8500 arthroplasties and found that patients with a BMI greater than 50 had an 18.3-fold increased risk of infection, while patients with a BMI between 40 and 50 had a 3.2-fold increased risk of infection compared to patients with a BMI less than 40.[12] Davis and colleagues followed up with over 1600 patients prospectively for 5 years after total hip arthroplasty and found that patients with a BMI greater than 35 had a 4.42-times higher rate of dislocation than those with a BMI less than 25 and found that these patients had increased rates of infection and poorer Harris Hip Scores and 36-Item Short Form Health Survey questionnaire (SF-36) scores.[13] Almost 300,000 patients undergoing primary total joint arthroplasty (TJA) were selected from the National Surgical Quality Improvement Program database and studied. An evaluation of these patients demonstrated increased rates of medical and surgical complications in obese patients. Patients with a BMI over 30 demonstrated increased infectious and medical complications while those with a BMI greater than 40 demonstrated longer operating times, length of stay, and higher rates of readmissions, reoperations, deep venous thrombosis, renal insufficiency, superficial infections, deep infections, and wound dehiscence.[14] Wagner and colleagues prospectively evaluated over 21,000 hips undergoing primary total hip arthroplasty and evaluated BMI as a continuous variable and its association with revision, dislocation infection, and common complications. They found that reoperation and implant revision or removal rates increased with increasing BMI and that increasing BMI was associated with increased rates of early hip dislocation, wound infection, and deep periprosthetic infection.[15] Evidence demonstrates not only increased rates of postoperative complications in the obese patient but also adverse impacts on postoperative limb alignment,[16] mechanical failure, failure after revision surgery,[17] as well as functional outcomes.[18,19] Obesity demonstrates inferior early and late functional results, Knee Society Scores, range of motion, and Western Ontario and McMaster Universities Osteoarthritis Index pain scores.[20]

Owing to the mounting evidence of increased complications in obese patients undergoing primary TJA, the American Association of Hip and Knee Surgeons Workgroup published an evidence-based statement on obesity in arthroplasty in 2011. They concluded that all obese patients, those with a BMI greater than 30, are at an increased risk of perioperative complications and that patients with a BMI greater than 40 are at a substantially increased risk of infection and revision. They recommended that strong consideration should be given to reducing weight and minimizing associated comorbidities (diabetes, hypertension, cardiac disease, obstructive sleep apnea, and malnutrition) prior to proceeding with elective joint-replacement surgery.[21] TJA in morbidly obese patients carries higher risk of perioperative morbidity and complications, and the plethora of literature demonstrating these risks has led many surgeons to adopt a strict BMI cutoff of 40 for patients undergoing TJA.[22]

CONCERNS REGARDING ACCESS TO CARE: BMI CUTOFFS

While strict BMI cutoffs have been used and endorsed, concern has been raised in the literature regarding whether these cutoffs are ethical or justifiable and if these cutoffs are limiting care to a vulnerable patient.[23] Evidence that raise the concern for the ethicality of BMI cutoffs includes an overall low absolute risk in comparison to other commonly accepted comorbidities, oversimplifying a preoperative risk assessment, concerns whether obesity is a truly modifiable risk factor, and concerns regarding which patient populations are predominantly affected by cutoffs.

Giori and colleagues evaluated nearly 30,000 joint arthroplasties and found that the odds ratio for major complications increased from 1.00 to 1.37 when BMI rises from 25 to 40. In absolute terms, the risk of major complications increased about 1.5%.[24] In contrast to this small increase in risk, Courtney and colleagues evaluated major complications in a cohort of total hip and knee arthroplasty patients and found much higher risks in common medical diagnoses.[25] They found that the odds ratio of a major complication was 9.71 in patients with congestive heart failure, 8.43 in patients with cirrhosis, 4.16 in patients with chronic obstructive pulmonary disease, and 2.8 in patients with coronary artery disease.[25] Additionally, Belmont and colleagues found that age greater than 80 years and an American Society of Anesthesiologists score > 2 are stronger risk factors for a major complication than BMI greater than 40, demonstrating odds ratios of 1.94 and 1.49, respectively.[26] Each of these risk factors demonstrated to be stronger than a BMI over 40 are diagnoses and risks that we commonly accept in joint-replacement surgery.

Evidence regarding an oversimplification of preoperative risk is supported by the fact that BMI does not account for variations in body composition, fat distribution, and the thought that risk does not abruptly jump with each subsequent change in BMI category. A population-based cohort study published by Abramowitz and colleagues demonstrated that the health effects of increased BMI are alleviated by increased muscle mass.[27] Several studies have additionally demonstrated that prepatellar fat thickness is a better predictor of complications than BMI in TKA.[28–30] Preoperative risk calculators have been created and published in the literature to attempt to address the oversimplification of preoperative risk based on BMI only by including other comorbidities and demographics in addition to BMI.[31–33]

While BMI and obesity is traditionally thought of as a modifiable risk factor, numerous studies raise concern about its reversibility in a majority of patients. Evidence has shown that an intensive outpatient weight-reduction program averages only about 8% body weight loss,[34] which may be possible for patients just over the BMI cutoff to begin with, but excludes a majority of patients. A study performed by Springer and colleagues evaluated the implications of withholding TJA in the morbidly obese patient and found that only 8% of patients denied surgery for a BMI greater than 40 eventually reach their BMI cutoff and undergo surgery.[35]

Finally, a study by Wang and colleagues evaluated nearly 22,000 adults in the NHANES and evaluated demographics, BMI cutoffs, and the odds of a joint-replacement surgery being performed.[23] They found that inflexible cutoffs with respect to BMI disproportionately discouraged hip and knee arthroplasty in vulnerable populations such as women, those of lower socioeconomic status, and non-Hispanic blacks.[23]

These concerns regarding access to care raise the question on whether BMI cutoffs should be used universally on a surgery that improves pain and function to avoid risks comparable to other commonly accepted risks and whether or not we are limiting patient care to at-risk populations.

ROLE OF BARIATRIC SURGERY AND TJA

Bariatric surgery is often used as a weight loss solution for the morbidly obese patient. Bariatric surgery can reduce BMI (on average 31%[36]) and improve diabetes, hypertension, hyperlipidemia, and sleep apnea.[37] The most common bariatric surgical procedures include open or laparoscopic banding, gastric sleeve, or Roux-en-Y bypass. As many arthroplasties have used strict BMI cutoffs, bariatric surgery has been explored as a way of reducing BMI, and therefore risk, in patients who are morbidly obese and unable to lose weight through other means.

For patients and surgeons that decide bariatric surgery may be the best option prior to TJA, there is evidence that a portion of these patients may never need a joint-replacement surgery. A randomized control study performed by Dowsey and colleagues found that over 30% of patients randomized to the intervention group and underwent bariatric surgery did not undergo TJA surgery due to symptomatic OA improvement with weight loss.[38] Evidence has also demonstrated an association between bariatric surgery and improved joint space width and KSS,[39] as well as knee musculoskeletal symptoms.[40–42]

For the past 20 years, the research has promoted the notion that bariatric surgery should be considered in the morbidly obese patient. Parvizi and colleagues demonstrated "excellent outcomes with an acceptable complication rate" in a small study of 20 patients who first received bariatric surgery prior to undergoing TJA.[36] Follow-up studies reporting decreased risk such as Kulkarni and colleagues helped guide surgeons to recommend bariatric surgery before arthroplasty because of significantly improved infection and readmission risk.[43] Werner and colleagues retrospectively evaluated morbidly obese patients who underwent bariatric surgery and compared them to those who did not undergo bariatric surgery among total knee patients.[44] They found that 90-day risks improved in patients who underwent bariatric surgery.[44] McLawhorn and colleagues reviewed the New York state database and determined that patients that had bariatric surgery prior to TJA had improved outcomes compared to matched morbidly obese patients.[45,46]

Over the past decade, as the patient population has continued to become more obese, and bariatric surgery more common,[47] the data have slowly begun to call into question previously good outcomes and, in some instances, demonstrate worse outcomes. Inacio and colleagues found that bariatric surgery may not provide dramatic improvement in postoperative surgical outcomes in TJA.[48] Li and colleagues published that bariatric surgery may improve short-term outcomes but not long-term outcomes in TJA patients.[49] Gu and colleagues performed a systematic review concluding that the literature remains conflicted on whether or not bariatric surgery improves TJA outcomes,[50] forcing surgeons to ask the following question: Does bariatric surgery prior to a TJA procedure improve outcomes or lead to worse outcomes?

The success of TJA relies upon the ability to maximize implant survivorship, minimize infection rates, and prevent all-cause revision. A 2018 retrospective review of Medicare patients found that compared to patients with metabolic conditions and without bariatric surgery, arthroplasty patients with previous bariatric surgery were 7.7-times (P = .038) more likely to suffer from an infection at 2 years than control.[51] In this same study, they determined that the risk of revision of TKA was 3.4-times greater (P = .003) than it was for those who did not undergo bariatric surgery. The largest retrospective study to date which included 2.7 million Medicare patients found that patients had prosthetic failure at a higher rate if they underwent bariatric surgery. Additionally, nearly all complications including death, implant failure, periprosthetic infection, and readmission were elevated in the bariatric surgery group.[52]

Given the currently published data demonstrating mixed efficacy in the ability of bariatric surgery to decreased risk in TJA, surgeon scientists have sought to evaluate if the time from bariatric surgery to TJA or type of bariatric surgery improves results. Parvizi and colleagues used the Healthcare Cost and Utilization Project California State Inpatient Database to identify over 300 total hip arthroplasties preceded by bariatric surgery and over 1000 TKAs preceded by bariatric surgery.[36] They found that patients who underwent arthroplasty more than 6 months after bariatric surgery were less likely to be readmitted within 90 days of their arthroplasty than those who underwent arthroplasty within 6 months of their bariatric surgery.[53] Sax and colleagues used a national, all-payer, database to elucidate if timing or type of bariatric surgery changed the risk profile in patients undergoing TJA.[54] They identified almost 2000 patients who underwent TKA between 6 months and 1 year after undergoing bariatric surgery and over 14,000 patients who underwent TKA more than 1 year after undergoing bariatric surgery. They further stratified these patients based on the type of bariatric surgery that they had performed, Roux-en-Y gastric bypass or sleeve gastrectomy. They also identified 2 comparison cohorts of patients who had not undergone bariatric surgery, one with a BMI greater than 50 and another with a BMI between 20 and 35. They found similar incidences of medical complications, surgical complications, and revisions in patients who underwent arthroplasty between 6 months and 1 year after bariatric surgery and those who underwent arthroplasty more than 1 year after bariatric surgery. Interestingly, they found no differences in complications based on the type of bariatric surgery performed (Roux-en-Y gastric bypass vs sleeve gastrectomy) and found that the comparison group with a BMI greater than 40 had greater medical and surgical complications and revisions than both bariatric surgery groups and the lower-BMI group.[54] Based on these data and risk profile, patients and surgeons should wait at least 6 months after bariatric surgery to proceed with TJA.

A RISK-STRATIFIED APPROACH

There is no doubt based on a plethora of evidence that obesity is related to increased complications in TJA. The rate of obesity in the

United States will only continue to rise, and it is estimated that the most common BMI category in the next 10 years will be "severe obesity" (BMI between 35 and 40). We know based on data published by Springer and colleagues that while obesity is extremely prevalent in the United States, it is even more prevalent among TJA patients.[35] This presents a unique problem for the orthopedic surgeon performing joint-replacement surgeries as the number of joint replacements will continue to rise, as will the prevalence of obesity.

While BMI cutoffs have previously been established to reduce risk, based on the evidence presented in this review, using strict BMI cutoffs may not be justified nor ethical when dealing with this at-risk population. BMI cutoffs may not represent a true preoperative risk assessment, and BMI in isolation has been shown to be a weak risk factor smaller than risk factors we commonly accept when performing joint-replacement surgery.[24–26] Additionally, while BMI is thought of as a modifiable risk factor, evidence has shown that it may only be reversible for a small subset of the population,[55] and by using BMI cutoffs, we are limiting care to vulnerable patient populations.[23]

It is our recommendation that a balanced approach be taken with regard to BMI and TJA. Owing to the increased risk of complications related to obesity and arthroplasty, every attempt should be made to modify the risk factor and achieve a BMI less than 40. If this is unable to be achieved despite great efforts, indicating that this risk factor is not reversible for the patient, an overall assessment of the patient's health should be considered. The surgeon and patient should optimize the medically controllable consequences of obesity such as diabetes, metabolic syndrome, hypertension, cardiac disease, obstructive sleep apnea, and malnutrition and ultimately have an informed discussion of risks and benefits when deciding whether to proceed.

SUMMARY

Obesity is a complex issue that needs to be addressed in TJA. Unfortunately, obesity will continue to rise, as will its complications associated with TJA. Orthopedic surgeons performing joint-replacement surgeries must be aware of the risks associated with obesity and make every attempt to modify the risk factor. BMI should be used in an overall assessment of the patient and their health when deciding to proceed with surgery rather than using strict BMI cutoffs.

REFERENCES

1. Adult Obesity Facts | Overweight & Obesity | CDC. Available at: https://www.cdc.gov/obesity/data/adult.html. Accessed 21 August, 2022.
2. Dietz WH. The response of the US Centers for Disease Control and Prevention to the obesity epidemic. Annu Rev Public Health 2015;36:575–96.
3. Ward ZJ, Bleich SN, Cradock AL, et al. Projected U.S. state-level prevalence of adult obesity and severe obesity. N Engl J Med 2019;381(25):2440–50.
4. Cao H. Adipocytokines in obesity and metabolic disease. J Endocrinol 2014;220(2):T47–59.
5. Steele CB, Thomas CC, Henley SJ, et al. Vital signs: trends in incidence of cancers associated with overweight and obesity - United States, 2005- 2014. MMWR Morb Mortal Wkly Rep 2017;66(39):1052–8.
6. How we estimated when obesity might catch smoking as the top cause of cancer - Cancer Research UK - Cancer news. Available at: https://news.cancerresearchuk.org/2018/09/24/how-we-estimated-when-obesity-might-catch-smoking-as-the-top-cause-of-cancer/. Accessed 21 August, 2022.
7. Alvarnas A, Alvarnas, Alvarnas J. Obesity and cancer risk: a public health crisis. Am J Manag Care 2019;25(11 Spec No):SP332–3. PMID: 31860246.
8. Hurt RT, Frazier TH, McClave SA, et al. Obesity epidemic: overview, pathophysiology, and the intensive care unit conundrum. JPEN J Parenter Enteral Nutr 2011;35(5 Suppl):4S–13S.
9. Reyes C, Leyland KM, Peat G, et al. Association between overweight and obesity and risk of clinically diagnosed knee, hip, and hand osteoarthritis: a population-based cohort study. Arthritis Rheumatol 2016;68(8):1869–75.
10. Odum SM, Springer BD, Dennos AC, et al. National obesity trends in total knee arthroplasty. J Arthroplasty 2013;28(8 Suppl):148–51.
11. Changulani M, Kalairajah Y, Peel T, et al. The relationship between obesity and the age at which hip and knee replacement is undertaken. Journal of Bone and Joint Surgery-British 2008;90-B(3):360–3.
12. Malinzak RA, Ritter MA, Berend ME, et al. Morbidly obese, diabetic, younger, and unilateral joint arthroplasty patients have elevated total joint arthroplasty infection rates. J Arthroplasty 2009 Sep;24(6 Suppl):84–8.
13. Davis AM, Wood AM, Keenan AC, et al. Does body mass index affect clinical outcome post-operatively and at five years after primary unilateral total hip replacement performed for osteoarthritis? A multivariate analysis of prospective data. J Bone Joint Surg Br 2011;93(9):1178–82.
14. Zusmanovich M, Kester BS, Schwarzkopf R. Postoperative complications of total joint arthroplasty in obese patients stratified by BMI. J Arthroplasty 2018;33(3):856–64.

15. Wagner ER, Kamath AF, Fruth KM, et al. Effect of body mass index on complications and reoperations after total hip arthroplasty. J Bone Joint Surg Am 2016;98(3):169–79.
16. Estes CS, Schmidt KJ, McLemore R, et al. Effect of body mass index on limb alignment after total knee arthroplasty. J Arthroplasty 2013;28(8 Suppl):101–5.
17. Watts CD, Wagner ER, Houdek MT, et al. Morbid obesity: increased risk of failure after aseptic revision TKA. Clin Orthop Relat Res 2015;473(8):2621–7.
18. Collins JE, Donnell-Fink LA, Yang HY, et al. Effect of obesity on pain and functional recovery following total knee arthroplasty. J Bone Joint Surg Am 2017;99(21):1812–8.
19. Deakin AH, Iyayi-Igbinovia A, Love GJ. A comparison of outcomes in morbidly obese, obese and non-obese patients undergoing primary total knee and total hip arthroplasty. Surgeon 2018;16(1):40–5.
20. Järvenpää J, Kettunen J, Soininvaara T, et al. Obesity has a negative impact on clinical outcome after total knee arthroplasty. Scand J Surg 2012; 101(3):198–203.
21. Workgroup of the American Association of Hip and Knee Surgeons Evidence Based Committee. Obesity and total joint arthroplasty: a literature based review. J Arthroplasty 2013;28(5):714–21.
22. Ricciardi BF, Giori NJ, Fehring TK. Clinical faceoff: should orthopaedic surgeons have strict BMI cut-offs for performing primary TKA and THA? Clin Orthop Relat Res 2019;477(12):2629–34.
23. Wang AY, Wong MS, Humbyrd CJ. Eligibility criteria for lower extremity joint replacement may worsen racial and socioeconomic disparities. Clin Orthop Relat Res 2018;476:2301–8.
24. Giori NJ, Amanatullah DF, Gupta S, et al. Risk Reduction Compared with Access to Care: Quantifying the Trade-Off of Enforcing a Body Mass Index Eligibility Criterion for Joint Replacement. J Bone Joint Surg Am 2018;100(7):539–45.
25. Courtney PM, Rozell JC, Melnic CM, et al. Who should not undergo short stay hip and knee arthroplasty? risk factors associated with major medical complications following primary total joint arthroplasty. J Arthroplasty 2015;30(9 Suppl):1–4.
26. Belmont PJ Jr, Goodman GP, Waterman BR, et al. Thirty-day postoperative complications and mortality following total knee arthroplasty: Incidence and risk factors among a national sample of 15,321 patients. J Bone Joint Surg Am 2014;96:20–6.
27. Abramowitz MK, Hall CB, Amodu A, et al. Muscle mass, BMI, and mortality among adults in the United States: a population-based cohort study. PLoS One 2018;13:e0194697.
28. Wagner RA, Hogan SP, Burge JR, et al. The radiographic prepatellar fat thickness ratio correlates with infection risk after total knee arthroplasty. J Arthroplasty 2018;33:2251–5.
29. Watts CD, Houdek MT, Wagner ER, et al. Subcutaneous fat thickness is associated with early reoperation and infection after total knee arthroplasty in morbidly obese patients. J Arthroplasty 2016;31: 1788–91.
30. Yu S, Siow M, Odeh K, et al. Periarticular soft tissue envelope size and postoperative wound complications following total knee arthroplasty. J Arthroplasty 2018;33:S249–52.
31. Bilimoria KY, Liu Y, Paruch JL, et al. Development and evaluation of the universal ACS NSQIP surgical risk calculator: a decision aid and informed consent tool for patients and surgeons. J Am Coll Surg 2013;217:833–42.
32. Bozic KJ, Ong K, Lau E, et al. Estimating risk in Medicare patients with THA: an electronic risk calculator for periprosthetic joint infection and mortality. Clin Orthop Relat Res 2013;471:574–83.
33. Harris AHS, Kuo AC, Weng Y, et al. Can machine learning methods produce accurate and easy-to-use prediction models of 30-day complications and mortality after knee or hip arthroplasty? Clin Orthop Relat Res 2019;477:452–60.
34. Unick JL, Beavers D, Bond DS, et al, Look AHEAD Research Group. The long-term effectiveness of a lifestyle intervention in severely obese individuals. Am J Med 2013;126:236–42.
35. Springer BD, Roberts KM, Bossi KL, et al. What are the implications of withholding total joint arthroplasty in the morbidly obese? A prospective, observational study. Bone Joint Lett J 2019;101B:28–32.
36. Parvizi J, Trousdale RT, Sarr MG. Total joint arthroplasty in patients surgically treated for morbid obesity. J Arthroplasty 2000;15(8):1003–8.
37. Buchwald H, Avidor Y, Braunwald E, et al. Bariatric surgery: a systematic review and meta-analysis. JAMA 2004;292(14):1724–37. Erratum in: JAMA. 2005 Apr 13;293(14):1728.
38. Dowsey MM, Brown WA, Cochrane A, et al. Effect of bariatric surgery on risk of complications after total knee arthroplasty: a randomized clinical trial. JAMA Netw Open 2022;5(4):e226722.
39. Abu-Abeid S, Wishnitzer N, Szold A, et al. The influence of surgically-induced weight loss on the knee joint. Obes Surg 2005;15:1437–42.
40. Hooper MM, Stellato TA, Hallowell PT, et al. Musculoskeletal findings in obese subjects before and after weight loss following bariatric surgery. Int J Obes 2007;31:114–20.
41. Chen SX, Bomfim FA, Youn HA, et al. Predictors of the effect of bariatric surgery on knee osteoarthritis pain. Semin Arthritis Rheum 2018;48(2):162–7.
42. Hacken B, Rogers A, Chinchilli V, et al. Improvement in knee osteoarthritis pain and function

following bariatric surgery: 5-year follow-up. Surg Obes Relat Dis 2019;15(6):979–84.
43. Kulkarni A, Jameson SS, James P, et al. Does bariatric surgery prior to lower limb joint replacement reduce complications? Surgeon 2011;9(1):18–21.
44. Werner BC, Kurkis GM, Gwathmey FW, et al. Bariatric surgery prior to total knee arthroplasty is associated with fewer postoperative complications. J Arthroplasty 2015;30(9 Suppl):81–5.
45. McLawhorn AS, Levack AE, Lee YY, et al. Bariatric surgery improves outcomes after lower extremity arthroplasty in the morbidly obese: a propensity score-matched analysis of a New York statewide database. J Arthroplasty 2018;33(7):2062–9.e4.
46. Arterburn D, Wellman R, Emiliano A, et al, PCORnet Bariatric Study Collaborative. PCORnet bariatric study collaborative. Comparative effectiveness and safety of bariatric procedures for weight loss: a PCORnet cohort study. Ann Intern Med 2018;169(11):741–50.
47. Estimate of bariatric surgery numbers, 2011-2020. American Society for Metabolic and Bariatric Surgery; 2022. Available at: https://asmbs.org/resources/estimate-of-bariatric-surgery-numbers.
48. Inacio MC, Paxton EW, Fisher D, et al. Bariatric surgery prior to total joint arthroplasty may not provide dramatic improvements in post-arthroplasty surgical outcomes. J Arthroplasty 2014;29:1359.
49. Li S, Luo X, Sun H, et al. Does prior bariatric surgery improve outcomes following total joint arthroplasty in the morbidly obese? J Arthroplasty 2019;34(3):577–85.
50. Gu A, Cohen JS, Malahias M-A, et al. The effect of bariatric surgery prior to lower-extremity total joint arthroplasty: a systematic review. HSS J 2019;15(2):190–200.
51. Lee GC, Ong K, Baykal D, et al. Does prior bariatric surgery affect implant survivorship and complications following primary total hip arthroplasty/total knee arthroplasty? J Arthroplasty 2018;33(7):2070–4.e1.
52. Meller MM, Goodman S, Gonzalez Mark H. Does bariatric surgery normalize risks after total knee arthroplasty? Administrative Medicare Data, JAAOS: Global Research and Reviews 2019;3(12):e1900102.
53. Schwarzkopf R, Lavery JA, Hooper J, et al. Bariatric surgery and time to total joint arthroplasty: does it affect readmission and complication rates? Obes Surg 2018;28(5):1395–401.
54. Sax OC, Chen Z, Bains SS, et al. Timing and type of bariatric surgery preceding total knee arthroplasty leads to similar complications and outcomes. J Arthroplasty 2022;37(8S):S842–8.
55. Shapiro JA, Narayanan AS, Taylor PR, et al. Fate of the morbidly obese patient who is denied total joint arthroplasty. J Arthroplasty 2020;35(6S):S124–8.

Managing the Patient with Peripheral Vascular Disease before Total Knee Arthroplasty Surgery

Andrew Fraval, MD, FRACS[a,*], William J. Hozack, MD[a]

KEYWORDS

• Total knee arthroplasty • Peripheral vascular disease • Vascular injury

KEY POINTS

- Peripheral vascular disease (PVD) is present in at least 2% to 4.6% of patients undergoing total knee arthroplasty (TKA), but is likely present in more.
- PVD can increase wound healing and infection complications after TKA and is an independent risk factor for arterial complications following TKA.
- An ankle-brachial index (ABI) is a helpful tool in determining the preoperative management strategies for patients with peripheral vascular disease undergoing TKA—consider a vascular consultation with a preoperative ABI of less than 0.9
- Vessel calcification seen on X-ray has been shown to be associated with high rates of tourniquet failure; however, there is inconclusive evidence for higher rates of complication associated with torniquet use in patients with vessel calcification.
- Patients with previous bypass graft surgery are at higher risk of vascular complication following TKA—consider a vascular consultation and not using a tourniquet.

INTRODUCTION

Peripheral vascular disease (PVD), defined as decreased arterial perfusion to the lower extremities due to atherosclerotic obstruction, is known to occur in patients undergoing total knee arthroplasty with described rates of between 2% and 4.5%[1–3] Our goal is to provide a comprehensive review of the pathophysiology of PVD as it relates to TKA, associated outcomes of patients undergoing TKA in the setting of PVD, diagnostic pearls, and current management strategies recommended in the published literature.

PATHOPHYSIOLOGY OF PERIPHERAL VASCULAR DISEASE

Peripheral vascular disease is primarily due to arthrosclerosis affecting the noncerebral and noncoronary arteries.[4] The sites of arthrosclerosis in the lower limb are usually the abdominal aorta, iliac, and femoral arteries although popliteal arteries may be affected. The atheroma consists of a core of cholesterol joined to proteins with a fibrous intravascular covering, the details of which are beyond the scope of this article.

The heterogeneous presentations of PVD have led to multiple classification systems described in the literature utilizing both clinical and radiological markers.[5] For the purposes of this review, The American College of Cardiology/American Heart Association (ACC/AHA) practice guidelines offer a useful system of classification, describing 4 categories for patients with PVD depending on their presentation.[6]

- Chronic, asymptomatic
- Chronic, with intermittent claudication (IC)
- Chronic with critical limb ischemia (CLI)

[a] Rothman Institute, Thomas Jefferson University, 925 Chestnut Street 5th Floor, Philadelphia, PA 19107, USA
* Corresponding author.
E-mail addresses: Andrew.Fraval@rothmanortho.com; afraval@mac.com

Orthop Clin N Am 54 (2023) 259–267
https://doi.org/10.1016/j.ocl.2023.02.011

- Acute limb ischemia (ALI)

In chronic PVD, which encompasses the first 3 categories, the arthrosclerotic plaque builds up slowly on the inside of arteries. In the early stages, the arteries compensate for the plaque buildup by dilating to preserve flow through the vessel. Eventually, the artery cannot dilate any further, and the atherosclerotic plaque starts to narrow the arterial lumen flow, leading to reduced tissue perfusion.

Asymptomatic PVD represents over 50% of patients with PVD with up to 70% of patients with asymptomatic PVD remain undiagnosed by the patient's primary care physician.[6] The majority of patients with underlying PVD presenting to an orthopedic surgeon for the consideration of a total knee arthroplasty would fit into this category.

Patients with intermittent claudication at rest compensate for significant stenosis via vessel dilation leading to decreased vascular resistance and increased flow. When mobilizing, the metabolic demands of the calf muscle increase, and there is insufficient blood flow to match those demands leading to muscle ischemia. This is the mechanism that leads to the characteristic symptoms of claudication, with aching pain typically in the calves and/or buttocks brought on by activity and relieved by rest.

Critical limb ischemia is defined as pain at rest or ulceration with or without tissue necrosis. Aggressive interventional treatment may be required to prevent limb loss. Usually, patients with critical limb ischemia present with an ankle-brachial (ABI) index less than 0.5 and toe systolic pressure less than 30 mm Hg.[7]

Acute limb ischemia may occur in the context of chronic PVD. This occurs when thrombi, emboli, or acute trauma compromises perfusion. Thrombus usually occurs due to plaque rupture and subsequent occlusive thrombus formation.[6] Regarding emboli, the femoral artery is the most common site, followed by the iliac arteries, aorta, and popliteal arteries.

The effect of a TKA on the underlying pathophysiology of PVD has been examined to some extent within the literature. One study by Dawson and colleagues investigated patients with no known diagnosis of PVD and found no effect of TKA on chronic limb ischemia, as measured by ankle-brachial indices (ABI).[8] Two studies examined the effects of TKA on lower limb blood flow in patients with a known background of PVD.[9,10] In both studies, TKA was performed using a tourniquet. Both studies measured ABIs pre and postoperatively and no changes occurred after surgery. These findings suggest that an uncomplicated TKA, despite the use of a tourniquet, has no negative impact on PVD in terms of reducing blood flow.

PREVALENCE OF PERIPHERAL VASCULAR DISEASE IN PATIENTS UNDERGOING TOTAL KNEE ARTHROPLASTY

A large cohort study of 1182 patients reported the overall prevalence of PVD in patients undergoing TKA as 2%.[1] Part of this cohort involved a prospective evaluation in which patients were reviewed by both orthopedic and vascular surgeons, supplemented with an ABI measurement as indicated. In this group, a prevalence of PVD of 7% was identified. This finding of higher rates when patients are screened carefully preoperatively is consistently reported in studies using a similar methodology. Another large series of 1000 patients, which prospectively examined patients scheduled for TKA with both an ABI and doppler sonography, found a prevalence of 4.6%.[3] Given patients with known PVD were excluded, the overall prevalence of PVD in the TKA patient population is undoubtably higher.

Smaller series of patients scheduled for TKA and examined with ABI and duplex have shown asymptomatic PVD to occur in up to 45% of patients.[10–12] One series of patients presenting to an orthopedic surgeon for the evaluation of lower extremity pain, when screened for a history of PVD including ABIs, was found to have a prevalence of PVD of 20%. In this same cohort, only 2% had symptomatic PVD.[13] In a recent nationwide database cohort study, 1,547,092 who underwent TKA were investigated for a diagnosis of PVD. In this cohort, the prevalence of PVD was 20%. This cohort was matched across relevant comorbidities including DM, hyperlipidemia, hypertension, and smoking status. This matching process may have elevated the prevalence in this cohort.[14]

Based on the published literature on the prevalence of PVD in patients undergoing TKA, it is clear that the rates of symptomatic or known PVD are low (around 2%–4%) but that undiagnosed asymptomatic PVD is present in substantially more patients.

IMPACT OF PERIPHERAL VASCULAR DISEASE ON TOTAL KNEE ARTHROPLASTY OUTCOMES

In a matched cohort analysis, Summers and colleagues[14] found that patients with PVD (as compared to controls patients without PVD) have longer inpatient stays (4 days vs 3 days), higher day of surgery and 90-day episode costs, higher 90-day readmission rates and higher rates of implant failure (Odds ratio of 1.41). Gad and colleagues[15] presented 94 patients with known PVD who underwent TKA. When this series was analyzed looking at patients with an ABI less than 0.7, there was a significantly higher hazard ratio for revision surgery as compared to patients with an ABI greater than 0.7.

Acute vascular injury following TKA is a rare but potentially devastating complication with a reported incidence of 0.03%–0.19%.[16–22] Peripheral vascular disease has consistently been found to be a risk factor for arterial injury associated with TKA[1,17,19,23–30] The mechanism for these injuries is usually indirect.[16,17,19,23] Vessels affected by artherosclerosis are more susceptible to mechanical stress which may lead to plaque rupture and subsequent thrombosis or embolis.[31] When revascularization is required in the postoperative setting, complications may be encountered including a reperfusion injury requiring prophylactic fasciotomies. When arterial complications associated with total knee arthroplasty do occur, they can be associated with additional serious complications such as infection, compartment syndrome, amputation, and even death due to overwhelming sepsis. The incidence of amputation, following a vascular complication associated with PVD is reported to be 20% to 64%.[2,30] A more recent systemic review found infection had overtaken PVD as the leading cause of amputation following TKA; however, still listed PVD as a significant risk factor.[32] The end result of any of these complications is a prolonged postoperative recovery associated with a worse functional outcome.

Peripheral vascular disease, with its accompanying decreased tissue perfusion, is an independent risk factor for prosthetic joint infection (PJI).[33] Delayed wound healing is also more common in patients that have undergone TKA and subsequently found to have decreased perfusion secondary to undiagnosed PVD.[34–36] In one series of patients requiring plastic surgery reconstruction for skin defects following chronic wound breakdown or infection, 67% were found to have pathologic vascular status.[34]

Medical complications have also been described as having an association with patients undergoing TKA with a diagnosis of PVD. An increased risk of acute perioperative cardiovascular events, postoperative anemia, increased postoperative blood transfusions, and urinary tract infections have all been shown to occur more frequently in patients with PVD following TKA.[14,37]

PATIENT EVALUATION

History

Some patients have a known history of PVD or previous vascular surgical intervention such as percutaneous transluminal angioplasty or bypass graft surgery at the time of presentation to their Orthopedic surgeon.

An occasional patient presents with pre-existing symptoms of intermittent claudication, classically described as a cramp in a muscle that affects the patients' ability to continue mobilizing and occurs at a reproducible distance when walking on a flat surface and is relieved quickly and consistently by rest.[38] The calves are the most common location for pain, with gluteal muscles being a less common site. Most commonly, symptoms present one joint below the stenosis causing a limitation of flow.[38] Symptoms of claudication should improve without the need to sit or adjust the position of the leg. This reflects the underlying cause as being a mismatch between metabolic demand and arterial flow, rather than a mechanical or compressive etiology as seen in knee osteoarthritis or neurogenic claudication. A careful enquiry as to the location and nature of the symptoms is necessary to delineate symptoms that may be associated with PVD as compared to those that arise due to knee osteoarthritis. Atypical symptoms in the setting of claudication may often be reported such as the leg feeling tired, giving way, or simply pain rather than the classic description of cramping.[39] Where claudication is suspected, a careful examination is warranted to differentiate a musculoskeletal from a vascular cause for the presentation.

Symptoms of ischemic pain at rest may also be present and represent critical limb ischemia. Pain at rest can occur in the setting of severe osteoarthritis and as such questions should be directed toward the location and quality of the pain to differentiate these etiologies.

Most patients who present for the consideration of TKA have *no* symptoms of PVD. As such, it is reasonable to assess risk factors to explore the possibility of asymptomatic PVD. Guidelines from the Trans-Atlantic Inter-Society Consensus (TASC), define increased risk for PAD as the presence of one or more of the following[40].

- Age less than 50 years with diabetes and one additional risk factor (smoking, dyslipidemia, hypertension, or homocysteinemia)
- Age 50 to 69 years with a history of smoking or diabetes
- Age $\geq$70 years

- Leg symptoms with exertion or ischemic rest pain
- Known coronary, carotid, or renal atherosclerosis
- Abnormal lower extremity pulses

Unfortunately, many patients being considered for TKA have at least one of the above risk factors. From a practical standpoint, in the absence of clinical symptoms of PVD, the most useful way to detect the presence of PVD is by physical examination.

Physical Examination

Examination should begin with inspection. Extremity ischemia alters the appearance of the skin. While changes in extremity appearance depend on the duration and severity of PAD, with diminished blood flow, the skin becomes thin dry, shiny, and at times hairless. Hair loss may not be a predictable indicator of PVD with mixed reports on this finding. In more severe PVD, ulcerations may occur typically located at the termination of arterial branches, commonly found on the tips of the toes and between the digits. Ischemic ulcers also form at sites of increased focal pressure, such as the lateral malleolus and metatarsal heads. The lesions often appear dry and punched out and are painful but exhibit little bleeding.[38]

Assessment and documentation of the pedal pulses is the most critical step in the evaluation of PVD in patients being scheduled for TKA. While not excluding the presence of PVD, palpable pedal pulses suggest sufficient circulation such that TKA can be performed safely. In the absence of palpable pedal pulses, we recommend further vascular examination starting with an ankle-brachial index (ABI).

Radiographic examination

Vascular calcifications, suggestive of PVD, are present in 4.1%–32% of patients undergoing TKA.[37,41,42] Of note, these patients can have normal pulses and no known history of PVD, making radiographic changes the only measure of identifying a patient as being at increased risk of complications.

Calcifications can be divided into 2 subtypes, intimal or medial,[43] based on radiographic appearance (Fig. 1). Intimal calcifications are atherosclerotic plaques in the intimal layer of the vessel wall, creating discrete, irregular, and patchy calcifications on X-ray. Medial calcification, also known as Moenckeberg's sclerosis, affects the tunica media and internal elastic lamina of the vessel wall, creating uniform, linear, parallel, track-like lines on X-ray. While intimal calcifications suggest the presence of PVD limiting blood flow, medial calcifications do not limit blood flow but do increase vessel rigidity.[44] These differing calcification patterns have implications with respect to intraoperative patient management as discussed later in discussion.

MANAGEMENT STRATEGIES

Ankle-brachial index (ABI)

While one indication for ABI is a patient who presents with clinical signs of ischemia as described above, the most common indication is a patient who does not have palpable pedal pulses (Fig. 2).

The resting ankle-brachial systolic pressure index (ABI) is a simple, well-studied test to evaluate the extent of PVD in patients undergoing TKA.[1–3,9,13,15,18,23,45] The ABI is a ratio of the ankle systolic blood pressure divided by the brachial systolic pressure detected with a Doppler probe.[46] It is an effective test at diagnosing PVD being highly sensitive (90%) and specific (98%).[47] An ABI from 0.9 to 1.3 excludes clinically significant arterial occlusive disease. An ABI of less than 0.90 has a high degree of sensitivity and specificity for PAD, using arteriography as the reference standard.[48] An ABI of 0.4–0.9 suggests a level of arterial obstruction sufficient to cause claudication, whilst an ABI less than 0.4 suggests critical limb ischemia. An ABI greater than 1.3 suggests the presence of noncompressible calcified vessels,[38] which may be visible on X-ray.

Most investigations into the effect of PVD on TKA have used the ABI as the measure of the severity of PVD and subsequent outcomes. De Laurentis and colleagues found an increased incidence of ischemic vascular complications when the ABI was less than 0.5[1]. Another study, evaluating patients with nonpalpable pulses planned for TKA, found no increased risk of vascular complications, even with abnormal ABIs as long as the femoral pulse was present and there was no skin ulceration or symptoms of rest pain.[9] In this small series of 73 patients, only 35 had ABIs less than 0.9 with the lowest recorded reading of 0.73. Bishoy and colleagues found a significant difference in reoperation following TKA prosthesis where an ABI was less than 0.7 as compared to greater than 0.9 in patients with known peripheral vascular disease. The reasons for reoperation included infection, loosening, and implant failure.

No prospective study has shown a difference in outcomes for patients with an ABI of 0.7 to 0.9

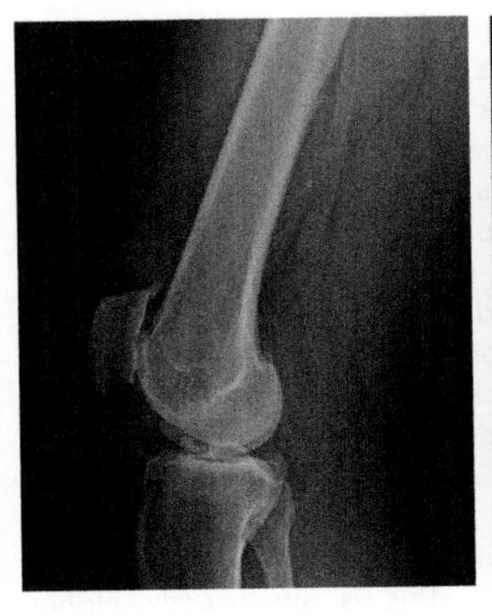

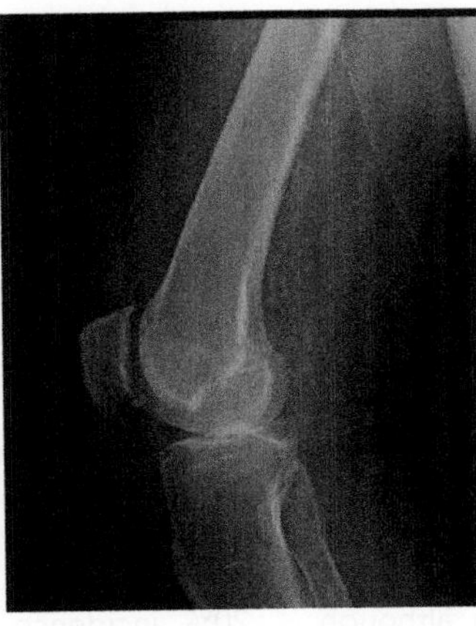

Fig. 1. Left: Medial calcifications seen as continuous, uniform, linear, parallel, track-like lines. Right: Intimal calcifications seen as discrete, irregular, patchy, plaque-like depositions of calcium.

and represents an area of uncertainty in terms of the safest course of action for the patients planned for TKA.

Finally, when no pedal pulses are palpable, a preoperative ABI can be useful as a baseline should any concern about limb vascularity arise postoperatively after TKA.

Vascular surgical consult

There are several suggested indications for preoperative vascular consultation. First, we recommend referral to a vascular surgeon prior to proceeding with surgery in those patients with any symptoms or signs of critical limb ischemia (claudication, rest pain, active arterial ulceration), A second indication for vascular consultation is for those patients with limb bypass surgery (see later in discussion). However, the most common reason is the presence of an abnormal ABI, recognizing that the indications for vascular surgical intervention (in the absence of acute ischemia) are not well-defined.

We do not recommend automatic vascular surgical preoperative consultation for patients with an established diagnosis of PVD. Most of these patients already have had vascular surgical consultation, and a phone call to that surgeon (as opposed to a formal consultation requiring a patient visit) is a reasonable approach.

Tourniquet use

In the setting of PVD, torniquet use in TKA has had mixed recommendations.

A recent Cochrane review recommended against the use of tourniquet citing higher rates

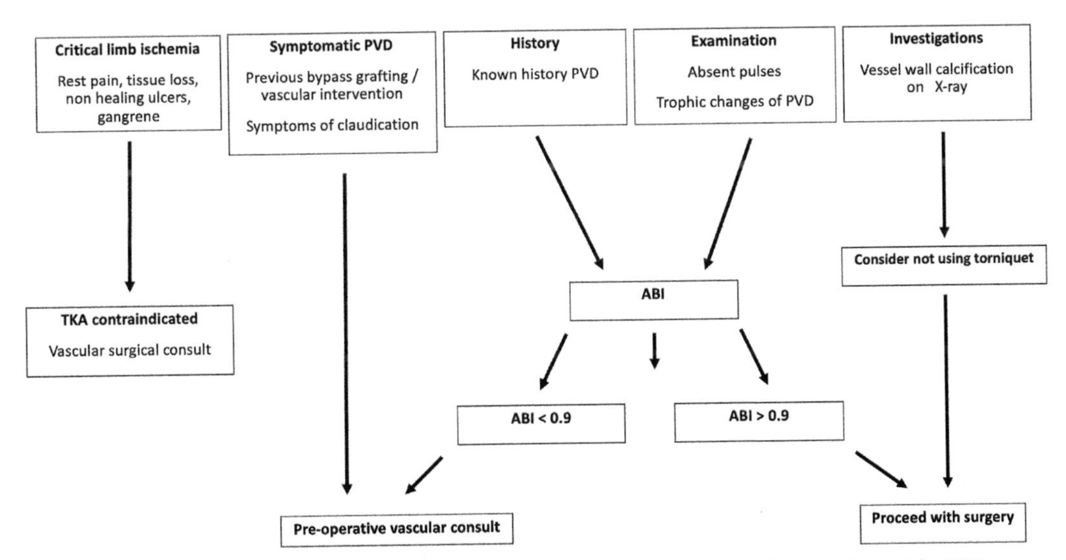

Fig. 2. A summary of the recommended management algorithm for patients with PVD planned for TKA.

of thromboembolic events, postoperative pain and longer inpatient stays without the benefit of decreased blood loss. In opposition to this, a recent well-designed prospective randomized controlled trial favored the use of tourniquet with reduced blood loss, improved visualization of surgical field, and range of motion.[49]

In the setting of vessel calcification, although not always due to PVD, there have been multiple reports of tourniquet failure leading to ineffective vascular compression and increased bleeding associated with vessel wall calcification. These studies mainly pertain to medial wall calcification where the arteries are less compressible than noncalcified vessels, although not associated with atherosclerosis.[15,41,50,51] Where intimal calcifications were present, representing atherosclerosis and PVD, tourniquet failure was not found to occur compared to patients without PVD.[52]

An association between vessel calcifications and arterial occlusion was made by Kobayashi and colleagues who reported that plaque disruption may occur due to the manipulation of the knee during TKA in patients with vessel calcification present on X-ray.[28] Due to this, they recommended against the use of tourniquet in the setting of calcifications which was further bolstered by publications in a similar time period.[1,22,53] Contrary to this recommendation is the finding by Koehler and colleagues who retrospectively reviewed a series of 373 patients who underwent TKA with the use of a tourniquet and found that vessel calcification did not increase the risk of vascular complications.[54] A further recent publication reporting on a series of 223, again failed to find an increased risk of complication following tourniquet use in patients with peripheral vascular disease.[41]

Vascular injuries following TKA are rare and, as such, firm conclusions can not be drawn from these relatively small series. Given the documented higher rates of tourniquet failure, and the literature to support safety of no tourniquet, our practice is to avoid tourniquet use in the setting of vascular calcifications (see Fig. 2).

Managing patients with previous bypass graft surgery

Patients planned for TKA with a history of previous bypass graft surgery present a particular challenge due to the documented risk of graft occlusion due to thrombosis following the procedure.[1,21,55,56,57] The incidence of a vascular complication following TKA in patients with in situ bypass graft is poorly described due to the rare nature of this event.

Given the rare occurrence of vascular injury following bypass graft surgery associated with TKA, the evidence available to formulate robust protocols is limited. De Laurentis and colleagues reported on this complication and recommended avoiding tourniquet use to minimize the chance of this occurring.[1] Dossche and colleagues reported on a single case of graft occlusion due to thrombosis following TKA where a tourniquet was not used and suggested that heparin intraoperatively may minimize the risk of thrombosis.[57] A series of 10 patients published by Turner and colleagues reported acute arterial occlusion in 2 patients representing a 20% incidence.[56] This is significantly higher than the overall rate of 0.03%–0.19%. The authors of this study recommended a protocol of preoperative graft evaluation using ultrasound to identify the presence of occult stenosis and the use of heparin to minimize thrombosis in addition to avoiding tourniquet use. A further single case report also described the use of heparin intraoperatively to minimize thrombosis; in this case, there was no injury to the graft. There are no comparative studies to support the protective effect of intraoperative heparin use or preoperative vascular studies.

In our institution, following extensive experience in managing patients with previous bypass graft surgery undergoing TKA, we have adopted the practice of a careful clinical evaluation of the patient to confirm the presence of pulses followed by proceeding to surgery without the use of a tourniquet. Avoiding the use of a tourniquet is recommended by all authors reporting managing patients with previous bypass graft surgery.[1,21,22,55–57] It is a reasonable consideration to seeking a vascular consult prior to surgery; however, our experience has been that where the graft is performing well clinically with the presence of pulses, the recommendation from vascular specialists is to proceed to surgery without the use of a tourniquet. It is also wise to inform patients regarding the possible increased risk of vascular complications as compared to a routine TKA.

SUMMARY

As outlined in this article, the presence of PVD is a known to affect the outcomes of TKA both in terms of the risk of complications as well as prosthesis survival. While the quoted incidence of PVD in patients undergoing TKA is relatively low, it is likely that up to 15% to 20% of patients have asymptomatic undiagnosed peripheral vascular disease. This highlights the importance of a thorough history and examination to screen for both symptoms and risk factors of PVD. An ABI is a simple office test that can be employed which informs the need for vascular referral prior to proceeding with surgery. Orthopedic surgeons should have a low threshold to conduct an ABI due to the documented higher complications associated with patients with an abnormal ABI undergoing TKA. Whilst the use of tourniquet in the setting of vascular calcifications is inconclusive, in the setting of previous bypass graft surgery, we recommend not to use a tourniquet. Any patient with critical limb ischemia as in the case of vascular ulcers needs a vascular consultation rather than a TKA.

DISCLOSURE

The authors have nothing to disclose.

REFERENCES

1. DeLaurentis DALK, Booth RE, Rothman RH, et al. Arterial and ischemic aspects of total knee arthroplasty. Am J Surg 1992;164(3):237–40.
2. Abu Dakka MBH, Al-Khaffaf H. Total knee arthroplasty in patients with peripheral vascular disease. Surgeon 2009;7(6):362–5.
3. Park IH, Lee SC, Park IS, et al. Asymptomatic peripheral vascular disease in total knee arthroplasty: preoperative prevalence and risk factors. J Orthop Traumatol 2015;16(1):23–6.
4. Peach G, Griffin M, Jones KG, et al. Diagnosis and management of peripheral arterial disease. BMJ Aug 14 2012;345:e5208. https://doi.org/10.1136/bmj.e5208.
5. Hardman RL, Jazaeri O, Yi J, et al. Overview of classification systems in peripheral artery disease. Semin Intervent Radiol 2014;31(4):378–88.
6. Conte SM, Vale PR. Peripheral Arterial Disease. Heart Lung Circ Apr 2018;27(4):427–32.
7. Campia U, Gerhard-Herman M, Piazza G, et al. Peripheral Artery Disease: Past, Present, and Future. Am J Med 2019;132(10):1133–41.
8. Dawson AG, Bachoo P, Sutherland AG. Does knee replacement surgery lead to chronic limb ischemia? J Knee Surg Dec 2010;23(4):223–8.
9. Bruce AS, Getty CJ, Beard JD. The effect of the ankle brachial pressure index and the use of a tourniquet upon the outcome of total knee replacement. J Arthroplasty Apr 2002;17(3):312–4.
10. Patil S, Allan DB, Quin R. Effect of total knee arthroplasty on blood flow to the lower limb: a prospective clinical study and review of literature. J Arthroplasty 2002;17(7):882–6.
11. Atilla HA. The prevalence of arterial and venous abnormalities in asymptomatic patients undergoing total knee arthroplasty. Turkish Journal of Vascular Surgery 2019;28(3):133–7.
12. Bowman NK, Appleyard M, Williams F, et al. The effect of total knee arthroplasty on lower limb blood flow. J Arthroplasty 2011;26(2):250–4.
13. Bernstein JEJ, Staska M, Reinhardt S, et al. The prevalence of occult peripheral arterial disease among patients referred for orthopedic evaluation of leg pain. Vasc Med 2008 Aug;13(3):235–8.
14. Summers S, Yakkanti R, Haziza S, et al. Nationwide analysis on the impact of peripheral vascular disease following primary total knee arthroplasty: A matched-control analysis. Knee Aug 2021;31: 158–63.
15. Gad BV, Langfitt MK, Robbins CE, et al. Factors influencing survivorship in vasculopathic patients. J Knee Surg 2020;33(10):1004–9.
16. Calligaro KD, Dougherty MJ, Ryan S, et al. Acute arterial complications associated with total hip and knee arthroplasty. J Vasc Surg 2003;38(6): 1170–5.
17. Parvizi J, Pulido L, Slenker N, et al. Vascular injuries after total joint arthroplasty. J Arthroplasty 2008; 23(8):1115–21.
18. Abularrage CJ, Weiswasser JM, Dezee KJ, et al. Predictors of lower extremity arterial injury after total knee or total hip arthroplasty. J Vasc Surg 2008; 47(4):803–7 [discussion: 807-8].
19. Troutman DA, Dougherty MJ, Spivack AI, et al. Updated strategies to treat acute arterial complications associated with total knee and hip arthroplasty. J Vasc Surg Oct 2013;58(4):1037–42.
20. Pal A, Clarke JM, Cameron AE. Case series and literature review: popliteal artery injury following total knee replacement. Int J Surg 2010;8(6): 430–5.
21. JA R. Vascular complications of total knee arthroplasty. Report of three cases. J Arthroplasty 1987; 2(2):89–93.
22. Calligaro KDDD, Booth RE, Rothman RH, et al. Acute arterial thrombosis associated with total knee arthroplasty. J Vasc Surg 1994;20(6):927–930doi.
23. Smith DE, McGraw RW, Taylor DC, et al. Arterial complications and total knee arthroplasty. J Am Acad Orthop Surg 2001;9(4):253–7.
24. Ko LJ, DeHart ML, Yoo JU, et al. Popliteal artery injury associated with total knee arthroplasty: trends, costs and risk factors. J Arthroplasty 2014; 29(6):1181–4.
25. Padegimas EM, Levicoff EA, McGinley AD, et al. Vascular complications after total knee arthroplasty-a single institutional experience. J Arthroplasty 2016;31(7):1583–8.
26. Matziolis G, Perka C, Labs K. Acute arterial occlusion after total knee arthroplasty. Arch Orthop Trauma Surg 2004;124(2):134–6.

27. Inomata K, Sekiya I, Otabe K, et al. Acute arterial occlusion after total knee arthroplasty: a case report. Clin Case Rep 2017;5(8):1376–80.
28. Kobayashi SIK, Koike T, Saitoh S, et al. Acute arterial occlusion associated with total knee arthroplasty. Arch Orthop Trauma Surg 1999;119(3–4): 223–224doi.
29. Park BJ, Cho HM, An KY, et al. Acute arterial occlusion following primary total knee arthroplasty. Knee Surg Relat Res 2018;30(1):84–8.
30. Garabekyan T, Oliashirazi A, Winters K. The value of immediate preoperative vascular examination in an at-risk patient for total knee arthroplasty. Orthopedics 2011;34(1):52.
31. Street MWJ, Howard LC, Neufeld ME, et al. Vascular injuries during hip and knee replacement. Orthop Clin North Am 2022;53(1):1–12.
32. Mousavian A, Sabzevari S, Ghiasi S, et al. Amputation as a complication after total knee replacement, is it a real concern to be discussed?: a systematic review. Arch Bone Jt Surg 2021;9(1):9–21.
33. Bozic KJ, Lau E, Kurtz S, et al. Patient-related risk factors for postoperative mortality and periprosthetic joint infection in medicare patients undergoing TKA. Clin Orthop Relat Res 2012;470(1):130–7.
34. Herold C, Steiert A, Knobloch K, et al. Angiographic findings in patients with postoperative soft tissue defects following total knee arthroplasty. Knee Surg Sports Traumatol Arthrosc 2011;19(12): 2045–9.
35. Ries MD. Skin necrosis after total knee arthroplasty. J Arthroplasty 2002;17(4 Suppl 1):74–7.
36. Zolper EG, Kotha VS, Walters ET, et al. Incidence of major arterial abnormality in patients with wound dehiscence after lower extremity orthopedic procedures. Plast Reconstr Surg 2020;146(6): 1382–90.
37. Cantu Morales D, de Beer J, Petruccelli D, et al. Lower extremity arterial calcification on preoperative knee radiographs as a predictor of postoperative cardiovascular events after primary total knee arthroplasty. J Arthroplasty 2018;33(4):1181–5.
38. Wennberg PW. Approach to the patient with peripheral arterial disease. Circulation 2013;128(20): 2241–50.
39. McDermott MMGP, Liu K, Guralnik JM, et al. Leg symptoms in peripheral arterial disease: associated clinical characteristics and functional impairment. JAMA 2001;286(13):1599–606.
40. Hirsch AT, Haskal ZJ, Hertzer NR, et al. ACC/AHA 2005 Practice Guidelines for the management of patients with peripheral arterial disease (lower extremity, renal, mesenteric, and abdominal aortic): a collaborative report from the American Association for Vascular Surgery/Society for Vascular Surgery, Society for Cardiovascular Angiography and Interventions, Society for Vascular Medicine and Biology, Society of Interventional Radiology, and the ACC/AHA Task Force on Practice Guidelines (Writing Committee to Develop Guidelines for the Management of Patients With Peripheral Arterial Disease): endorsed by the American Association of Cardiovascular and Pulmonary Rehabilitation; National Heart, Lung, and Blood Institute; Society for Vascular Nursing; TransAtlantic Inter-Society Consensus; and Vascular Disease Foundation. Circulation 2006;113(11):e463–654.
41. Yoo JH, Kim JG, Chung K, et al. Vascular calcification in patients undergoing total knee arthroplasty: frequency and effects on the surgery. Clin Orthop Surg 2020;12(2):171–7.
42. Woelfle-Roos JV, Dautel L, Wernerus D, et al. Vascular calcifications on the preoperative radiograph: predictor of ischemic complications in total knee arthroplasty? J Arthroplasty 2016;31(5):1078–82.
43. Jinnouchi H, Sakamoto A, Torii S, et al. Types and pathology of vascular calcification. Coronary Calcium 2019;1–25.
44. Sucker C, Lanzer P. Arteriosclerosis and media sclerosis. A comparison of 2 calcifying vascular diseases. Medizinische Klinik (Munich, Germany: 1983) 2000;95(4):207–10.
45. Li Z, Xiang S, Bian YY, et al. Diagnosis and treatment of arterial occlusion after knee arthroplasty: the sooner, the Better. Orthop Surg 2019;11(3):366–72.
46. Grenon SM, Gagnon J, Hsiang Y. Ankle–Brachial Index for Assessment of Peripheral Arterial Disease. N Engl J Med 2009;361(19):e40.
47. Doobay AV, Anand SS. Sensitivity and specificity of the ankle-brachial index to predict future cardiovascular outcomes: a systematic review. Arterioscler Thromb Vasc Biol 2005;25(7):1463–9.
48. 3rd ME. Peripheral arterial disease: identification and implications. Arch Intern Med 2003;163(19):2306–14.
49. Goel R, Rondon AJ, Sydnor K, et al. Tourniquet use does not affect functional outcomes or pain after total knee arthroplasty: a prospective, double-blinded, randomized controlled trial. J Bone Joint Surg Am 2019;101(20):1821–8.
50. Agrawal A, Arora A, Srivastava AK, et al. Use of tourniquet during knee arthroplasty in patients with radiographic arterial calcifications. J Arthroplasty 2020;35(8):2050–3.
51. Barr LIU, Sardesai A, Chitnavis J. Tourniquet failure during total knee replacement due to arterial calcification: case report and review of the literature. J Perioper Pract 2010;20(2):55–8.
52. Woelfle-Roos JV, Dautel L, Mayer B, et al. Vascular calcifications on the preoperative radiograph: harbinger of tourniquet failure in patients undergoing total knee arthroplasty? Skeletal Radiol 2017; 46(9):1219–24.

53. Kumar SNCJ, Rawlins I. Vascular injuries in total knee arthroplasty. A review of the problem with special reference to the possible effects of the tourniquet. J Arthroplasty 1998;13(2):211–216doi.
54. Koehler SMFA, Noori N, Weiser M, et al. Safety of tourniquet use in total knee arthroplasty in patients with radiographic evidence of vascular calcifications. Am J Orthoped 2015;44(9):E308–16.
55. Maruyama Y, Ochiai T, Kobayasi S, et al. Total knee arthroplasty after an artificial femoral-popliteal arterial bypass graft. Eur J Orthop Surg Traumatol 2009;19(8):595–8.
56. Turner NS 3rd, Pagnano MW, Sim FH. Total knee arthroplasty after ipsilateral peripheral arterial bypass graft: acute arterial occlusion is a risk with or without tourniquet use. J Arthroplasty 2001; 16(3):317–21.
57. Dossche L, Brabants KA. Arterial graft occlusion after total knee arthroplasty treated by prompt thrombectomy. J Arthroplasty 2002;17(5):670–2.

Socioeconomic Challenges in the Rural Patient Population in Need of Total Joint Arthroplasty

Aaron Sesler, BS, Jeffrey B. Stambough, MD,
Simon C. Mears, MD, PhD, Charles Lowry Barnes, MD,
Benjamin M. Stronach, MS, MD*

KEYWORDS

- Total joint arthroplasty • Rural health care • Socioeconomic factors
- Social determinants of health • Health-care inequalities

KEY POINTS

- Rural patients have less access to primary care and even less access to surgical specialists, creating a subset of patients who endure higher costs, poorer outcomes, and difficulty in getting total joint arthroplasty.
- Improved pathways of care may help rural systems to develop streamlined ways to optimize patients for total joint arthroplasty.
- Innovation in telehealth may help to decrease disparities of care in rural populations.
- Future studies should focus on delineating the reasons for discrepancies in total joint arthroplasty underutilization of rural patients and in promoting methods to improve utilization equality.

INTRODUCTION

Total joint arthroplasty (TJA) is a high-volume procedure with nearly 2 million procedures performed annually in the United States.[1,2] Despite progress in arthroplasty, racial and socioeconomic disparities persist, particularly regarding patient access to care.[3] Rural patients have unique challenges regarding access to and utilization of resources for health care. This is due to a combination of factors including lack of access to local specialized care, isolated living requiring long distance travel, and reticence in seeking care. Longer life expectancies in an aging population and improvement of arthroplasty implants have all broadened the utility of TJA[4,5] but health-care inequalities in the rural population remain.[3,6,7] In addition, age, socioeconomics, and regional distribution all play an important role in access to orthopedic services.[6] This review provides a framework to better understanding current challenges facing rural patients in need of arthroplasty care.

RURAL HEALTH CARE

The term "rural" has widely been accepted as relating to characteristics of the country or country life, with strong ties to agriculture and functional independence.[8] "Rural," as defined by the United States (US) Office of Management and Budget in 1993 comprises, "all areas outside a metropolitan area,"[9] with 72% of the US land area qualifying as rural. Despite the majority of the US landmass being rural, only 59.5 million people (19%) of the US population reside in a

Department of Orthopaedic Surgery, University of Arkansas for Medical Sciences, 4301 West Markham Street Mail, Little Rock, AR 72205, USA
* Corresponding author. Department of Orthopaedic Surgery, University of Arkansas for Medical Sciences, 4301 West Markham Street Mail Slot #531, Little Rock, AR 72205.
E-mail address: bstronach@uams.edu

Orthop Clin N Am 54 (2023) 269–275
https://doi.org/10.1016/j.ocl.2023.02.012
0030-5898/23/

rural area according to the US Census bureau data.[10,11] In present society, there are multiple definitions of "rural" with no currently accepted single definition with the term often referring to a geographic location within a state or region, along with describing individuals who live in sparsely populated areas. This often leads to variability when capturing the size of rural populations. For example, The US Department of Agriculture estimates there are 46 million rural Americans (14%), which is in contrast to the Census Bureau data estimate of 59.5 million rural residents (18%).[10,12] Danek and colleagues further concluded that the geographic units and definitions to determine rurality were used inconsistently within and across multiple studies.[12]

There is also debate as to the definition of a rural hospital. The American Hospital Association (AHA) defines rural hospitals as those not located within a metropolitan area.[13] Rural and urban hospitals differ in many categories such as facilities, charges per discharge, length of stay, and location distribution.[14] There are 1805 rural hospitals located in the United States as of 2019 with 47% of these hospitals having 25 or less inpatient beds and are categorized as critical access hospitals (CAH). This hospital designation was created by the Medicare Rural Hospital Flexibility Program of the 1997 Balanced Budget Act in an effort to increase resources for small, geographically isolated hospitals, many of which were struggling financially.[15,16] Hospitals that converted to CAH status became eligible for cost-based, rather than diagnosis related group–based, reimbursement.[16] CAH facilities continue to face many challenges with the lack of clinical and technological resources, poorer performance metrics, and higher mortality rates than non-CAHs. This is further complicated by CAHs being exempt from the 2010 Affordable Care Act quality improvement and standards. Almost half of CAHs have experienced financial problems, which have been exacerbated by the COVID-19 pandemic, and elimination of safety-net services has led to widespread hospital closures, further decreasing access to care in rural communities.[16–18] Furthermore, when a rural hospital closes, residents often experience an average increase in travel time of 30 minute to the nearest hospital.[16,19] Additionally, travel distance has been identified as the greatest barrier to seeking health care as identified by 33% of older rural patients,[20,21] with hospital closures adding to this barrier to care. The AHA data regarding hospital closures from 2015 to 2019 places the future of care in rural communities in grave danger as rural hospitals shut down at a higher rate.[22]

The Institute of Medicine describes health-care quality as the "degree to which health services for individuals and populations increase the likelihood of desired health outcomes and are consistent with current knowledge."[23] Little is known about measuring quality in rural medical care, particularly rural medical procedural care, where relatively small numbers of procedures are performed by generalists. Sustainability of rural hospitals and equipment is also a concern. Providers may struggle to keep appropriate staffing levels, maintain a broad scope of technical skills, and purchase modern tools and equipment. In addition, new trained professionals seem to be increasingly unavailable to ease the current workforce demands, let alone to replace those retiring or withdrawing from services.

The number of citizens living below the poverty line is disproportionately higher in rural areas, yet the number of rural residents on Medicaid is lower. Urban patients receive 20% to 30% more medical services than do rural residents. Most researchers identify rural areas as those with a relatively low population density and, within such an area, the number of providers tend to be below average with the practice population dispersed over a wide area.[24] Rural communities have disproportionately fewer health-care providers with 15% of physicians and less than 10% of general surgeons practicing in rural areas.[25] Local-area primary care physician supply is similar in rural and metropolitan areas but specialist supply is 31% lower in rural areas with fewer patients having any contact with a specialist.[9,26] There is a need for rural physicians to have a wide spectrum of practice capabilities due to fewer available providers that would be more reflective of a provider in the midtwentieth century. It is common for primary care physician may also provide obstetric and gynecologic care.[9] A general surgeon would be able to perform basic otolaryngologic and orthopedic procedures. As medical training has increasingly become subspecialized and expertise has become more focused, training structures have moved in the opposite direction for what may be best suited for rural providers who could best serve their patients with broader training. There also remains a need for common surgical procedures requiring specialized training, such as arthroplasty, to be provided in rural hospitals. Proposals to help address this need include the development of residencies and fellowships dedicated to training surgeons who are interested in practicing in rural areas, networking with university tertiary care hospitals, equal pay for equal work, liability reform, and regionalization of rural surgery centers so multiple surgeons can work as a team so that lifestyle and travel issues can be addressed.[9]

DISPARITIES IN CARE BASED ON PATIENT LOCATION

Disparities in utilization of TJA have been strongly linked to gender, race, and socioeconomic status (SES).[27] Multiple socioeconomic factors are associated with disparities in TJA access, including lower education levels, lower income, and significant comorbidities being associated with decreased TJA rates.[4,27–29] However, less information exists regarding utilization of TJA because it relates to disparities in the urban versus rural populations. Despite a high demand for orthopedic care in rural populations, there is scarce literature that details the access and outcomes of surgical interventions within these communities. Patients from these underserved areas often have higher medical comorbidities and require greater resource utilization to access orthopedic health care.[6,30] Community-level disadvantages affect the rate of TJA utilization in rural communities even when controlling for gender, racial, ethnic, and distance-to-hospital variabilities.[31] Many potential candidates for THA or TKA require health optimization by their surgeon for comorbidities such as tobacco use, obesity, malnutrition, diabetes, congestive heart failure, and kidney disease.[4,29,32] This process can be quite onerous for patients in rural areas, which places their quality care at risk.[33] Neuburger and colleagues found that, on average, patients living in socioeconomically deprived areas had worse outcomes after a hip or knee arthroplasty in part due to having worse health and more severe joint disease before treatment.[34] Kamath and colleagues found that TJA patients living in rural areas were more likely to be non-White, of Hispanic ethnicity, obese, current smokers, and had lower levels of education.[3] Furthermore, it was noted in a large cohort study involving elective patients with THA in Pennsylvania that patients from low area deprivation index level communities were more likely to be discharged to an institution as opposed to home for postoperative care and rehabilitation.[3,31]

Rural location is increasingly being recognized as an indicator of deprivation and poorer patient outcomes, which represents a dimension of disparity in health care.[3] There is limited data available on the influence of area-based deprivation regarding TJA utilization[3,35] but patients living in socioeconomically deprived areas had worse outcomes after surgery due to poor preoperative health status, increased disease severity, and less postoperative improvement in comparison to patients in socioeconomically stable communities.[34] Further research is needed to better understand the specific role of rural versus urban location in regards to access to care from the lens of socioeconomically deprived areas.

COMORBIDITIES

Social determinants of health (SDHs) describe the external factors that affect personal perspectives of health and are grouped into fixed domains to include economic stability, education access and quality, health-care access and quality, neighborhood environment and community support.[36] SDH significantly affects the cost and availability of health care in underserved communities. Many diseases are highly correlated to poor SDH, including obesity, cardiovascular disease, and smoking, which disproportionately affect rural populations.[4,29] Thirty five percent of the American population is considered obese (body mass index [BMI] $>$ 30). Furthermore, obesity is associated with postoperative complications, including wound complications, infections, and need for revision surgery.[4,37] Food security plays an important and complex role in nutritional status, and 10.5% of American households are currently food insecure, more of which are located in rural communities.[4]

Social deprivation is defined as a disconnection from healthy social and interpersonal relationships and is measured utilizing the social deprivation index, which has been correlated with population health outcome measures.[38] Few studies have investigated the influence of social deprivation on the costs and outcomes of patients undergoing TJA. However, Barrack and colleagues analyzed patient satisfaction and outcomes following TKA and determined that incomes of less than US$25,000 in deprived areas were less likely to be satisfied with surgical outcomes, more likely to have functional limitations such as postoperative pain and had increased disability after TKA than patients with higher incomes.[6]

SDHs, such as living in an impoverished area, significantly affect the ability for patients to have access to TJA due to total cost of care. Clement and colleagues found, when assessing for social deprivation as being a key factor for advanced arthritis, that the patients with more comorbidities and lack of education underwent surgery at an earlier age, were more likely to be women, to have more comorbidities and to suffer worse pain and function.[39] Social deprivation is also thought to be an etiologic factor for osteoarthritis of the knee, and according to assessments of pain and function, these patients have an increased need for TJA, in turn creating additional costs.[39,40] The association of rural location and its effect on social deprivation is not well understood and warrants further investigation because it relates to health-care access.

FINANCES

Overall costs to provide arthroplasty care have increased, which places added financial stress on CAH facilities. The average actual hospital expense for total knee arthroplasty increased from US$10,122 in 1983 to US$22,837 in 2013.[41,42] There is an associated increase in expenses for hospital systems based on geographic location, with rural areas being more impacted than urban centers. In an effort to control cost and standardize care, multiple health-care organizations, including Medicare, private insurers, and hospital systems, have enacted cost containment efforts for TJA procedures in the form of bundled care.[41] The margins for profit in arthroplasty have narrowed as bundled care has sought to contain costs and penalize certain outcomes. This can pose a significant barrier to smaller hospitals with low arthroplasty volumes and is a concern for access to TJA care in rural communities with patients having to seek out care in metropolitan areas that can be quite a long distance away from their community. Furthermore, patients with lower SES have been shown to utilize more resources in the 90-day episode of care. Including patient geographic and SES status to risk adjustment models may help avoid potential problems with access to joint arthroplasty care.[43]

Rural patients often make up the lowest income quartiles, around US$39,000 to US$47,999, contributing to a large income discrepancy when compared with urban counterparts at US$63,300. Additionally, lower SES often correlates to labor-specific jobs and increased risk for musculoskeletal injury. Review of current literature suggests that knee disorders due to occupation primarily consist of bursitis, meniscal lesions or tears, and osteoarthritis. Example industries include mining, construction, manufacturing, and custodial services where knee-bending postural activities exist as a commonality.[44] Specifically for TJA, lower income in rural patients has been associated with an increased risk for revision surgery, higher 30-day and 90-day readmission rates, unplanned surgery for surgical site infection, experiencing prosthetic hip dislocations or wound complications, and extended length of stay compared with the higher earning urban cohort.[2] Because of their association with higher comorbid burden, for these reasons, rural patients have higher cost surrounding the episode of TJA care. After adjusting for SES, one study found that ethnic minorities and low household income were associated with longer length of stay after TJA in patients in rural areas.[30] Improved pre-TJA optimization may allow for better outcomes in rural populations.

OPTIMIZATION OF RURAL HEALTH CARE

Remote Health is defined by Wakerman as an emerging discipline with distinct sociologic, historical and practice characteristics, further distinguished by geographic, professional and, often, social isolation of practitioners.[45] A strong multidisciplinary approach, team members of various roles, practitioners requiring public health, emergency and extended clinical skills all enhance the optimization of rural health care. Such optimal utilization of patient health care depends on the careful balance between the disease presence, access to care for that disease, the effective utilization of resources, and strategies for optimizing health-care access for specific patient populations. Factors such as socioeconomics, demographics, preoperative level of function, preoperative disease state, and geographic location all play important roles in the availability of proper access to specialized care such as orthopedics. Some simple tools for optimization in rural patients include assessing for food security, knowledge of a social safety net and community resources, patient diabetic literacy, and relationships with primary care providers to ensure routine communication to check up on patients. This can also minimize postoperative complications from diagnosed diabetes.[46] Optimization of TJA within rural areas depends on programs that have been implemented to hold sustainable access to care and allow for proper resources for their respective patient populations. O'Conner and colleagues noted strategies for optimization through a holistic assessment of the patient's nutritional status, further including metrics such a BMI greater than 18.5 kg/m^2, vitamin D level greater than 30 ng/dL, albumin level greater than 3.5 g/dL, transferrin level greater than 200 mg/dL, and TLC of greater than 1500 cells/mm^3.[29] One abnormal metric of malnutrition can predispose a patient to poor perioperative outcomes. Thus, identifying patients with malnutrition should be accomplished early through screening for food security, including geographic and resource-oriented ability to procure healthy food. Patients with identified undernutrition through positive screenings and surveys can also be referred to a nutritionist or weight-management specialist. Rehabilitation services such as occupational therapy, physical therapy, and speech-language therapy can be delivered via telehealth. The use of telehealth to supplement care increased rates of patient satisfaction for therapy services delivered to rural communities.[47,48]

SUMMARY

Optimizing TJA in the rural patient population depends on factors such as deprivation, education, employment, household income, and access to proper surgical institutions. Rural individuals have less access to primary care and even less access to surgical specialists, creating a distinct subset of patients who endure higher costs, poorer outcomes, and lack of care. Moreover, socioeconomic burden, comorbidities, and inability to access surgical specialists leads to the underutilization of TJA. Urban teaching and nonteaching hospitals continue to see equivalent proportional growth, which outpaced TJA volume growth of rural hospitals. Reducing SES disparities in health will require policy initiatives addressing the components of SES (income, education, and occupation) as well as the pathways by which these affect health. With advancements in remote patient technologies, telehealth/digital health may offer appealing solutions for rural patients to improved offer the potential for timely addressing of modifiable risk factors. Future studies should be focused on further delineating the reasons for these discrepancies in TJA underutilization of rural patients and methods of improving utilization equality should be explored.

CLINICS CARE POINTS

- Only 19% of the US population lives in a rural area despite 72% of the US landmass being rural.
- Living in a rural setting represents a disparity in access to healthcare with unique challenges when seeking care.
- Remote health strategies are being developed to improve the quality of care for rural communities in an effort to improve overall health of the rural population.

DISCLOSURE

The authors have nothing to disclose.

REFERENCES

1. Shah KC, Poeran J, Zubizarreta N, et al. Comparison of total joint arthroplasty care patterns prior to the Covid-19 pandemic and after resumption of elective surgery during the Covid-19 Outbreak: A retrospective, large urban academic center study. Knee 2022;38:36–41.
2. Kremers HM, Larson DR, Crowson CS, et al. Prevalence of total hip and knee replacement in the United States. Journal of Bone and Joint Surgery - American 2014;97(17):1386–97.
3. Kamath CC, O'Byrne TJ, Lewallen DG, et al. Association of rurality and neighborhood level socioeconomic deprivation with perioperative health status in total joint arthroplasty patients: analysis from a large, tertiary care hospital. J Arthroplasty 2022;37(8):1505–13.
4. Sabesan VJ, Rankin KA, Nelson C. Movement is life—optimizing patient access to total joint arthroplasty: obesity disparities. J Am Acad Orthop Surg 2022;30(21):1028–35.
5. Palazzuolo M, Antoniadis A, Mahlouly J, et al. Total knee arthroplasty improves the quality-adjusted life years in patients who exceeded their estimated life expectancy. Int Orthop 2021;45(3):635–41.
6. Barrack RL, Ruh EL, Chen J, et al. Impact of socioeconomic factors on outcome of total knee arthroplasty knee. Clin Orthop Relat Res 2014;472:86–97. Springer New York LLC.
7. Dixon T, Shaw M, Ebrahim S, et al. Trends in hip and knee joint replacement: Socioeconomic inequalities and projections of need. Ann Rheum Dis 2004;63(7):825–30.
8. Gessert C, Waring S, Bailey-Davis L, et al. Rural definition of health: a systematic literature review. BMC Publ Health 2015;15(1):378.
9. Shively EH, Shively SA. Threats to rural surgery. Am J Surg 2005;190(2):200–5.
10. Ratcliffe M, Burd C, Holder K, et al. Defining Rural at the U.S. Censusu Bureau; 2016. Available at: http://www2.census.gov. Accessed January 20, 2023.
11. Story map series. mtgis. Available at: https://mtgis-portal.geo.census.gov/arcgis/apps/MapSeries/index.html?appid=49cd4bc9c8eb444ab51218c1d5001ef6. Accessed January 15, 2023.
12. Danek R, Blackburn J, Greene M, et al. Measuring rurality in health services research: a scoping review. BMC Health Serv Res 2022;22(1):1340.
13. Fast facts: U.S. rural hospitals infographic: AHA (no date) American Hospital Association. Available at: https://www.aha.org/infographics/2021-05-24-fast-

facts-us-rural-hospitals-infographic. Accessed January 20, 2023.
14. Hatten JM, Connerton RE. Urban and rural hospitals: how do they differ? Health Care Financ Rev 1986;8(2):77–85.
15. Casey M, Moscovice I, Hung P, et al. 2012. Critical access hospital year 7 hospital compare participation and quality measure report. (Flex monitoring Team Briefing paper no.31). Available at: http://www.flexmonitoring.org/documents/Hospital-CompareReport-Year7.pdf. Accessed January 20, 2023.
16. Baernholdt M, Keim-Malpass J, Hinton ID, et al. A comparison of quality of care in critical access hospitals and other rural hospitals. Online J Rural Nurs Health Care 2014;14(2):3–31.
17. Holmes GM, Pink GH, Friedman SA. The financial performance of rural hospitals and implications for elimination of the Critical Access Hospital program. J Rural Health 2013;29(2):140–9.
18. Rhodes JH, Santos T, Young G. The early impact of the COVID-19 pandemic on hospital finances. J Healthc Manag 2023;68(1):38–55.
19. Fleming ST, Williamson HA, Hicks LL, et al. Rural hospital closures and access to services. Hosp Health Serv Adm 1995;40(2):247–62.
20. Goins RT, Williams KA, Carter MW, et al. Perceived barriers to health care access among rural older adults: a qualitative study. J Rural Health 2005; 21(3):206–13.
21. Buzza C, Ono SS, Turvey C, et al. Distance is relative: unpacking a principal barrier in rural healthcare. J Gen Intern Med 2011;26(Suppl 2):648–54.
22. American Hospital Association homepage: AHA (2023) American Hospital Association. Available at: https://www.aha.org/. Accessed January 15, 2023.
23. Allen-Duck A, Robinson JC, Stewart MW. Healthcare quality: a concept analysis. Nurs Forum 2017; 52(4):377–86.
24. Cox J. Rural general practice in the United Kingdom. Occas Pap R Coll Gen Pract 1995;71: 1–49. v-vii.
25. Sariego J. Patterns of surgical practice in a small rural hospital11No competing interests declared. J Am Coll Surg 1999;189(1):8–10.
26. Johnston KJ, Wen H, Joynt Maddox KE. Lack of access to specialists associated with mortality and preventable hospitalizations of rural medicare beneficiaries. Health Aff 2019;38(12):1993–2002.
27. Chisari E, Yayac M, Sherman M, et al. Which socioeconomic factors affect outcomes following total hip and knee arthroplasty? J Arthroplasty 2021; 36(6):1873–8.
28. Rahman R, Canner JK, Haut ER, et al. Is Geographic Socioeconomic Disadvantage Associated with the Rate of THA in Medicare-aged Patients? Clin Orthop Relat Res 2021;479(3):575–85.
29. O'Connor MI, Bernstein J, Huff T. Movement is life—optimizing patient access to total joint arthroplasty: malnutrition disparities. J Am Acad Orthop Surg 2022;30(21):1007–10.
30. Keeney BJ, Koenig KM, Paddock NG, et al. Do aggregate socioeconomic status factors predict outcomes for total knee arthroplasty in a rural population? J Arthroplasty 2017;32(12):3583–90.
31. Banerjee D, Illingworth KD, Novicoff WM, et al. Rural vs. urban utilization of total joint arthroplasty. J Arthroplasty 2013;28(6):888–91.
32. Urish KL, Qin Y, Li BY, et al. Predictors and cost of readmission in rotal knee arthroplasty. J Arthroplasty 2018;33(9):2759–63.
33. Litwic A, Edwards MH, Dennison EM, et al. Epidemiology and burden of osteoarthritis. Br Med Bull 2013;105(1):185–99.
34. Neuburger J, Hutchings A, Black N, et al. Socioeconomic differences in patient-reported outcomes after a hip or knee replacement in the English National Health Service. J Publ Health 2013;35(1): 115–24.
35. Sheth MM, Morris BJ, Laughlin MS, et al. Lower socioeconomic status is associated with worse preoperative function, pain, and increased opioid use in patients with primary glenohumeral osteoarthritis. J Am Acad Orthop Surg 2020;28(7):287–92.
36. Social Determinants of Health (no date) Social Determinants of Health - Healthy People 2030. Available at: https://health.gov/healthypeople/priority-areas/social-determinants-health. Accessed January 15, 2023.
37. Kremers HM, Visscher SL, Kremers WK, et al. The effect of obesity on direct medical costs in total knee arthroplasty. J Bone Joint Surg 2014;96(9):718–24.
38. Butler DC, Petterson S, Phillips RL, et al. Measures of social deprivation that predict health care access and need within a rational area of primary care service delivery. Health Serv Res 2013;48(2pt1):539–59.
39. Clement ND, Jenkins PJ, Nie YX, et al. Socioeconomic status affects the Oxford knee score and Short-Form 12 score following total knee replacement. Bone Joint Lett J 2013;95-B(1):52–8.
40. Schroer WC, Diesfeld PJ, LeMarr AR, et al. Modifiable risk factors in primary joint arthroplasty increase 90-day cost of care. J Arthroplasty 2018;33(9):2740–4.
41. Healy WL, Rana AJ, Iorio R. Hospital economics of primary total knee arthroplasty at a teaching hospital. Clin Orthop Relat Res 2011;469:87–94. Springer New York LLC.
42. Healy WL, Finn D. The hospital cost and the cost of the implant for total knee arthroplasty. A comparison between 1983 and 1991 for one hospital. J Bone Joint Surg 1994;76(6):801–6.

43. Courtney PM, Huddleston JI, Iorio R, et al. Socioeconomic risk adjustment models for reimbursement are necessary in primary total joint arthroplasty. J Arthroplasty 2017;32(1):1–5.
44. Reid CR, Bush PM, Cummings NH, et al. A review of occupational knee disorders. J Occup Rehabil 2010;20(4):489–501.
45. Wakerman J. Defining remote health. Aust J Rural Health 2004;12(5):210–4.
46. Wiznia DH, Jimenez R, Harrington M. Movement is life—optimizing patient access to total joint arthroplasty: diabetes mellitus disparities. J Am Acad Orthop Surg 2022;30(21):1017–22.
47. Harkey LC, Jung SM, Newton ER, et al. Patient satisfaction with telehealth in rural settings: a systematic review. Int J Telerehabilitation 2020;12(2):53–64.
48. What works? Strategies to improve rural health (no date) County Health Rankings & Roadmaps. Available at: https://www.countyhealthrankings.org/reports/what-works-strategies-improve-rural-health. Accessed January 20, 2023.

Pediatrics

Friends Not Foes

Optimizing Collaboration with Subspecialists

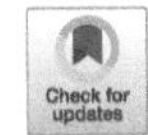

Nathaniel G. Rogers, MD[a,*],
Maria Carrillo-Marquez, MD[b], Annette Carlisle, MD[c],
Catherine D. Sanders, MD[d], Lauren Burge, MD[e]

KEYWORDS

- Subspecialist consultation • Preoperative planning • Comanagement • Child abuse
- Pediatric hospital medicine

KEY POINTS

- Refer for preoperative consultations well in advance of scheduling surgery and consider sending high-risk patients for nutrition assessment.
- Consider consulting a subspecialist perioperatively as early as possible for any patient with complex medical needs.
- When collaborating with a subspecialist, communication is key. It is imperative from the beginning of the collaboration to the end to have effective, clear communication regarding the clinical question and treatment recommendations.
- Pediatric infectious diseases consultation is recommended for patients with suspected or confirmed acute or chronic musculoskeletal infection in order to intervene acutely, establish a plan for disease surveillance and monitor for potential adverse effects of antibiotic therapy.
- There are specific evidence-based criteria regarding appropriate imaging for the diagnosis and screening of child physical abuse.

In the United States, the concept of using a multidisciplinary approach between surgical and medical specialties has been dated back to World War II, when field hospitals were utilized to care for soldiers. Since then, multidisciplinary teams have been established in various fields including burn, long-term rehabilitation, and surgery.[1] A multidisciplinary approach utilizing various specialties, including hospitalists and subspecialists, has been shown to positively affect patient care.[2] In this article, we aim to review key considerations for optimizing collaboration with pediatric subspecialists in the management of pediatric orthopedic patients.

For the purposes of this article, we define key roles as follows:

Primary team: The hospital team responsible for admitting the patient and providing primary intervention(s). This consists of the day-to-day care for the patient, including placing orders, following up on interventions, and making discharge plans.

Consultant: As defined by the Joint Commission, a licensed independent practitioner (LIP) is one "who has been asked to evaluate a patient and provide consultation, by way of an order from another LIP. The findings are entered into the medical record and may be used by other

[a] Division of Pediatric Hospital Medicine, University of Tennessee Health Science Center, 49 North Dunlap Street, Memphis, TN 38103, USA; [b] Division of Infectious Diseases, University of Tennessee Health Science Center, 49 North Dunlap Street, Memphis, TN 38103, USA; [c] Division of Allergy & Immunology, University of Tennessee Health Science Center, 49 North Dunlap Street, Memphis, TN 38103, USA; [d] Division of Pulmonology, University of Tennessee Health Science Center, 49 North Dunlap Street, Memphis, TN 38103, USA; [e] Division of Child Abuse, University of Tennessee Health Science Center, 49 North Dunlap Street, Memphis, TN 38103, USA
* Corresponding author.
E-mail address: nroger10@uthsc.edu

Orthop Clin N Am 54 (2023) 277–285
https://doi.org/10.1016/j.ocl.2023.02.002

practitioners to determine the ongoing course of care, treatment, or services."[3]

Management of pediatric orthopedic patients can occur using different models. In the traditional consultation model, the primary team (orthopedics) consults the subspecialist with the expectation that the consultant will provide recommendations to the team. The primary team will then consider the recommendations and carry out recommendations they deem appropriate.[4] This model differs from a comanagement model, which the Society of Hospital Medicine defines as the "shared responsibility, authority, and accountability for the care of a hospitalized patient...[where] the surgeon manages surgery related treatments, and a hospitalist manages the patient's medication conditions."[5]

Numerous studies have demonstrated the advantage of utilizing multidisciplinary comanagement. A study by Simon, and colleagues reported that medically complex pediatric spinal fusion patients, who were comanaged by both the orthopedic surgeon and hospitalist, had a decrease length of hospital stay.[6] Similarly, Rohatgi, and colleagues demonstrated a decrease in medical complications, length of stay (LOS), and cost of care in both orthopedic and neurosurgery patients that followed a surgical comanagement model.[7] Rapport and colleagues showed that medically complex children undergoing spinal fusion surgery benefit from comanaged teams led by hospitalists, requiring fewer days of parenteral nutrition and fewer laboratory studies.[2] Additionally, a survey of pediatric and orthopedic subspecialties found that although few participants thought that comanagement with hospitalists improved length of hospital stay or pain management, surgical subspecialties did view comanagement with hospitalists as having a positive impact on comorbidity management and care coordination.[8]

Whether collaboration with a subspecialist is warranted should be evaluated on a case-by-case basis. Comanagement with a subspecialist should be considered in those with a complex medical history, those with comorbid conditions, or those with a current condition that is outside of the primary team's scope of practice and/or comfort level. Common examples of comorbidities an orthopedist may encounter include cerebral palsy, prematurity, genetic syndromes, and poorly controlled asthma. These patients may benefit from early collaboration and/or comanagement with subspecialists as part of presurgery planning as well as ongoing support after surgery. Examples of subspecialists one may wish to engage include child abuse pediatrics if there is a question regarding the mechanism of injury or concern for possible abuse, infectious disease (ID) for recommendations regarding interoperative cultures or antibiotic regimens as well as transition of care to the outpatient setting, and Pediatric Hospitalist (PH) Medicine to manage comorbid conditions while the patient is hospitalized. If collaboration and/or comanagement with a subspecialist is required, consider involving the subspecialist as early as possible, either as an outpatient referral before surgery or at the onset of hospital admission. This allows the subspecialist needed time to adequately delve into the patient's unique history and recommend appropriate management plans. Other considerations for optimizing collaboration include clarifying the specific clinical question(s) the subspecialist should address, noting the urgency of the consult, and communicating after consultation between the primary and consulting team to discuss the recommendations and make contingency plans. Perhaps, most importantly when collaborating with subspecialists, it is essential for both parties to have an ongoing and clear communication both verbally as well as documented in the patient's chart.[9]

PREOPERATIVE PLANNING

Preoperative planning and medical management of comorbid conditions are essential aspects in the care of a child requiring a scheduled orthopedic intervention. Children with complex medical conditions, including cerebral palsy, neuromuscular disease, genetic syndromes, and sequelae of premature birth frequently require surgical invention for orthopedic problems, particularly, spinal deformities. These conditions, as well as other medical comorbidities, such as diabetes mellitus, put patients at higher risk of postoperative spinal surgery complications, including surgical site infections, prolonged mechanical ventilation, pneumonia, and readmission following hospital discharge.[10–15] Thus, advanced planning for spinal surgery or other orthopedic interventions is recommended.

There is currently limited guidance for preoperative management of comorbidities ahead of orthopedic surgery in children in the medical literature and few studies exploring the efficacy of multidisciplinary preoperative care in reducing surgical complications. Miller and colleagues demonstrated improvements in total hospital LOS, pediatric intensive care unit

(PICU) LOS, and number of days intubated in a matched case series in children undergoing spinal surgical interventions for neuromuscular scoliosis after the implementation of a preoperative care pathway involving multiple pediatric subspecialists.[16] A similar study by Visser, and colleagues, however, showed no difference in postsurgical complications with the use of a standardized, multidisciplinary preoperative protocol.[17] More research is therefore needed to better assess the optimal model for preoperative medical planning, and a standardized approach may not prove to be the best model in a patient population with such varied and complex needs.

Which patients should be referred to subspecialists for evaluation and to which subspecialists should they be referred before an orthopedic intervention?

Children who are already followed by a subspecialist for a medical condition, including diabetes mellitus, asthma, cystic fibrosis, seizure disorder, a neuromuscular condition, renal disease, rheumatologic disease, or sickle cell disease, should be assessed by their subspecialist for disease control and readiness for surgery *before* scheduling the operation. A thorough medical history and review of systems should be undertaken to assess the need for new referrals to subspecialists.

Special consideration for preoperative medical assessment is recommended in patients undergoing spinal procedures, particularly those with neuromuscular scoliosis. Neuromuscular disease, including muscular dystrophy, cerebral palsy, spinal muscular atrophy, spina bifida, and other genetic causes of hypotonia, is a significant risk factor for complications after spinal surgery, including prolonged need for mechanical ventilation, prolonged PICU LOS, pneumonia, and hospital readmission following discharge.[11–13,15] Limited mobility, poor cough clearance, restrictive lung impairment, obstructive sleep apnea, and/or chronic respiratory insufficiency/failure may contribute to these outcomes, and referral to a pediatric pulmonologist is recommended to assess for these risk factors and optimize respiratory status. In those with other causes of scoliosis, including idiopathic, thoracic curvatures greater than 70° may predict restrictive impairment and necessitate a preoperative pulmonology evaluation.[18]

How Far in Advance Should a Patient Be Referred to a Subspecialist?

Because of clinic scheduling wait times and time necessary to evaluate, treat, and optimize any medical condition, the surgical team should consider requesting patient appointments with their established subspecialist(s) at least 6 months ahead of the anticipated surgery date and with new subspecialist(s) 9 to 12 months ahead of the anticipated surgery date.

What Might a Preoperative Assessment Include?

Although each subspecialist assessment will entail a different approach to the evaluation and treatment of comorbidities, the pulmonology assessment of a patient ahead of spinal surgery exemplifies what an assessment might include.

Prentice and colleagues describe the role of a preoperative evaluation in a patient with a spinal deformity, which includes defining the effect the spinal deformity on lung function and/or the airway anatomy, assessing for gas exchange abnormalities, and anticipating any perioperative pulmonary issues.[19] Evaluation may include imaging studies (chest x-ray or computed tomography scan), pulmonary function testing (PFT), polysomnogram, blood gas, and/or exercise testing. Note that PFT may not be feasible in children who are aged younger than 6 years or developmentally delayed or in those with limited mobility or a tracheostomy. Interventions may include initiation/optimization of inhaled therapies, initiation/optimization of airway clearance therapies, surgical intervention to address obstructive sleep apnea, and/or initiation/optimization of positive airway pressure.

Should Patients Undergoing an Orthopedic Intervention Have a Preoperative Nutrition Evaluation?

Adequate nutrition is necessary for normal growth and development in children and carries even greater import during periods of physiologic stress, such as the perioperative period. Studies consistently demonstrate an increase in adverse postoperative events in children with abnormal nutrition (both undernutrition and overnutrition), including children with cerebral palsy undergoing spinal surgery.[20–23] Thus, preoperative nutrition assessment and invention is recommended to address a patient's nutritional needs.[24] Although a recent retrospective study did not show improvement in postoperative complication rates in children with cerebral palsy who underwent nutritional assessment before derotational osteotomy, the study does not specify how far ahead of surgery the assessment was completed, what type of nutritional intervention/rehabilitation was performed, and whether there was adequate time between the assessment and the surgery date for the interventions to be effective.[25] Because nutritional interventions and rehabilitation can require significant periods to be effective, it is recommended that a nutrition evaluation be performed at least 6 months ahead of the anticipated surgery date.

Perioperative Collaboration

Child maltreatment

Why is accurate identification of child maltreatment important to the orthopedic surgeon? Child abuse and neglect is encountered frequently by orthopedists, with fractures acting as a leading presentation for physical abuse.[26] Around 42% of these fractures are deemed definite or likely abusive and often act as an entry point for further evaluation of the child and family.[27] Once a child has been identified to be at risk for abuse or neglect, additional services or interventions may be offered, ideally to promote child health and safety. The risk of not recognizing child abuse may result in further injury to the child, escalation of injury, permanent disability, or even death. One study demonstrated that one-third of children with healing abusive fractures had previous medical visits where the diagnosis of abuse was not recognized, and these children most commonly had signs of trauma (bruising) at the previous visits.[28] Recognizing and reporting child abuse is thus a crucial concern for the orthopedic surgeon.

What is a child abuse pediatrician (CAP)? Child abuse pediatrics (CAP) has been an official pediatric subspecialty since 2006, and CAPs are now required to complete a 3-year fellowship and a board examination.[29] CAPs have special training in the recognition, diagnosis, prevention, reporting, and research of child abuse and neglect. Many large medical centers and children's hospitals have a CAP on faculty; however, some rural or suburban hospitals may not have access to a trained child protection team. These teams are usually led by a CAP and may also consist of a social worker, nurse, or nurse practitioner, and possibly a sexual assault nurse examiner. CAPs are ideally positioned to identify mimics of child physical abuse. Bleeding disorders, bone disease, endocrine abnormalities, and genetic illnesses are just a few of the medical entities that may mimic findings seen in child maltreatment, and with the help of other subspecialists, the CAP may guide the medical team through appropriate diagnostic channels and steer away from a detrimental incorrect diagnosis of abuse.

When should a child abuse pediatrician be consulted? A CAP may be consulted any time a physician or health-care professional has concern for child abuse or neglect. However, as mandated reporters themselves, orthopedists may not think a consult with a CAP is necessary if the reported injury is simple, well-documented, or witnessed by multiple observers. For example, if a 5-year-old child reports to an emergency room with a spiral fracture of the left tibia after bouncing off a trampoline onto the grass below while playing at a family picnic, the orthopedic provider would likely recognize that the mechanism provided is consistent with the given injury, the child is fully mobile, and developmentally able to complete the alleged injurious activity. The provider can therefore feel confident that the likelihood of abuse is low in this context, and no further workup is needed. However, should a case present with nuanced historical variations, multifactorial trauma mechanisms, and/or intrinsic medical illnesses that may influence a specific injury presentation, the particular skills of a CAP would be best suited to evaluate the case. Such cases may also be expected to present in the judicial system, and often orthopedic providers do not relish spending time testifying in a courtroom. A CAP, however, has training and experience in cogently and effectively translating medical information to case workers, attorneys, judges, and juries to present the medical facts of the child's injuries, medical prognosis, and probability of abuse optimally and accurately.

The level of concern for abuse is not always equally shared or highly correlated among child protection workers, child abuse pediatricians, and other physicians. Having early and frequent involvement of a CAP could prove beneficial because these decisions frequently have significant clinical and medical-legal implications.[30] It is also important to keep in mind that involving a CAP may also keep families from being falsely accused by spending the time and using their expertise in providing alternate diagnosis when appropriate and rendering their medical opinion to aid in Child Protective Services investigation. In many cases, non-CAP physicians may not have the time, training, or resources to offer optimal care to the allegedly abused child or be fully equipped to guide investigations. It has been reported that in cases in which there was concern for child physical abuse, there was disagreement surrounding the final diagnosis between CAP and non-CAP physicians in 42% of these cases. In 81% of these cases, CAPS indicated *less* concern for abuse than their non-CAP peers, again illustrating the importance of offering the most complete medical evaluations by the most qualified physicians to children who are reported to be abused or neglected.[31] The best approach is for orthopedists and child protection teams to work in concert, allowing the frequent exchange of information and offering a mutually collaborative medical impression that provides a united and clear medical diagnosis for the benefit of the child and investigatory agencies.

Difficult conversations

The orthopedic surgeon's first responsibility is to recognize child maltreatment, and then to report it to the appropriate agencies. Orthopedic surgeons may hesitate to disclose to families their concern for possible maltreatment; however, open and honest communication is foundational to maintaining a therapeutic relationship with the family. The surgeon should describe that reporting to government agencies is standard of care for every child with these specific injuries and to not report would be negligent and possibly criminal. The physician should disclose to caretakers that a report has been made with clear and concise language without inference of guilt. The physician should also appropriately recognize any limitations regarding the current medical information or future investigatory or criminal proceedings.[32–34]

Transferring the patient to another facility does not negate the orthopedic surgeon's obligation to report concerns of abuse to the appropriate agencies. If a CAP is also participating in the care of the abused child, it is paramount that the orthopedist supports the CAP in the diagnosis of abuse when speaking to the family or caretakers individually or to investigatory agencies. If the orthopedist does not agree with the CAP's conclusion, then both medical teams should meet to discuss their difference in diagnosis and an optimal approach to discussing medical plans to the family moving forward to minimize confusion and inconsistency.

Pediatric hospital medicine

What is an ideal orthopedic patient for a pediatric hospitalist to see? A pediatric hospitalist (PH) is trained in general pediatrics and focuses on acute care medicine of hospitalized children. Their patient demographics range from newborn babies to adults with congenital diseases. PHs are experienced in comanaging complex patients with both surgical and medical subspecialists. In addition to providing general pediatrics education to students and housestaff, they often sit on hospital and administrative committees, thus, offering an understanding of how hospital systems affect patient care.

Although a PH can see any admitted patient, studies show that increasing a PH census may lead to unnecessary laboratory test and subspecialist consultation.[33] The American Academy of Pediatrics (AAP) recommends PH consultation for any patient admitted to the hospital whose attending does not have experience in treating pediatric patients.[35] Specifically, AAP recommends a PH consultation if your patient is aged younger than 14 years, less than 40 kg in weight, medically complex or projected to exceed 24-hour LOS.

For example, a teenager with no medical problems being observed overnight after elective surgery may not require a PH consultation. Additionally, preoperative risk evaluation by a PH is typically not indicated, although a preoperative subspecialist consultation may be warranted depending on your patient's comorbidities.

How does pediatric hospitalist consultation affect your patient's care directly? If there are plans to consult a PH, it is preferred to be consulted as early during the hospital course as possible. This gives the PH a better understanding of the chronicity, severity, and clinical course of the patient's medical problems. This is of great importance as the overinvolvement of subspecialists may lead to an increase in health-care costs or prolonged hospital stay without changing the patient's overall hospital or clinical course.[36] Multiple studies have shown that PH can decrease LOS (up to almost 30%) particularly for complex patients without adversely affecting patient care.[37] Additionally, given their experience with patients of all chronologic ages and development, PHs have been shown to recognize pain more effectively, especially in preverbal patients.[38] As such, PHs are familiar with medication formulations, weight-based dosing, medication flavoring, and age-appropriate guidelines of specific medications. Finally, as physicians specifically trained to recognize and treat acute medical illness, PHs are skilled in identifying and formulating appropriate and cost-effective interventions early in the hospital admission. To achieve these ideal outcomes, the PH will need to follow the patient early in the hospital course.

How does pediatric hospitalist consultation affect the health-care institution directly? Health-care institutions value high standards of care and cost-effective medicine. Health-care administration sees the value in reduced LOS that PH can help maintain.[34] Additionally, patient and family satisfaction has also been shown to be higher when PHs are involved.[35] Beyond patient care, PHs are typically very accessible thereby increasing direct communication between nursing and physician staff. This not only improves nursing satisfaction—and ultimately nursing retention—but also streamlines treatment when acute medical problems develop.[38]

When should primary team consult a subspecialist over a pediatric hospitalist? A PH is trained in managing both chronic and acute medical problems. If an acute medical problem develops or a chronic medical problem flares, the primary service has the choice to consult a generalist or specialist. In general, it is reasonable to consult with a PH with any acute change in a patient's medical condition. The PH may determine whether he or she feels comfortable managing the medical problem or if a subspecialist would be better suited to care for the patient's specific medical problem. It is worth noting, if a specific medical comorbidity is in exacerbation on admission or is expected to worsen during the patient's hospital course, it is reasonable to discuss the utility of a subspecialist consultation on admission. Again, if there is uncertainty surrounding the need for a subspecialist consultation, a PH and an orthopedist may collaborate in establishing the most appropriate care for the patient.

Infectious diseases consultation

One of the most common reasons for pediatric infectious diseases (ID) specialist consultation are skin and soft tissue infection (SSTI) and musculoskeletal infections (hematogenous, traumatic, or surgical associated osteomyelitis, myositis and pyomyositis, septic arthritis, and so forth), which are also common entities for which orthopedic care is needed.[39]

ID specialists are familiar with the local antibiogram and the ever-evolving resistance patterns of common causative microorganism for osteoarticular infection and can help determine thresholds for choice of empirical antibiotic therapy, which are largely based on expert opinion.[40] ID also helps in identifying the best available definitive antibiotic therapy based on microbiological diagnosis.

Pediatric ID specialists play a role in the inpatient setting by consulting with the primary care physician on treatment of patients with complex conditions, offering evidence-based recommendations on diagnosis and management and optimize treatment by recommending appropriate antibiotic choice, duration, route of administration and by conducting therapeutic drug monitoring, when indicated, and by assessing for adverse drug reactions. ID specialists also facilitate transition of care to the outpatient setting by providing management and oversight of oral or IV antibiotics.[41]

Numerous studies in adults and children have evaluated the "value" of the ID consultation in patient care.[42] ID involvement has been associated to increased frequency of correct diagnosis,[43] shorter LOS,[44] more appropriate and fewer antibiotics used overall[45,46] but specifically in patients with trauma, SSTI,[47] bacteremia,[48] and bone and joint infections.[49] Another study found significant lower mortality, readmissions, shorter hospital and ICU LOS, and lower health-care costs in adult patients who received early ID interventions, specifically within 2 days of admission, which emphasizes the importance of early ID consultation.[50]

Staphylococcus aureus is the most common cause for SSTI and musculoskeletal infections in children,[51] and ID consultation for the management of patients with *S aureus* bacteremia is recommended because improvement in patient outcomes has been demonstrated when ID is involved.[48,52]

Orthopedic surgeons and ID specialists have a long history of collaboration. One example is the recently published guidelines by the Pediatric Infectious Diseases Society of America and Infectious Diseases Society of America for the management of acute hematogenous osteomyelitis, which were developed by a panel of experts in pediatric ID, general pediatric, pediatric emergency medicine, pediatric orthopedic surgery, and epidemiology. The guidelines have been reviewed and approved by the Pediatric Orthopedic Society of North America. Similar guidelines for septic arthritis are also in progress. One of the major take away points from the guidelines is the strong recommendations to transition patients to an oral antibiotic regimen rather than outpatient parental antibiotics, an appropriate and well-tolerated antibiotic option is available, and the patient has shown a response to an initial IV antimicrobial therapy.[51] Earlier transitions to oral therapy have been reported for the treatment of bone and joint infections in children after ID consultation service was implemented.[53]

CLINICS CARE POINTS

- Refer for preoperative consultations well in advance of scheduling surgery and consider sending high-risk patients for nutrition assessment.
- Consider consulting a subspecialist perioperatively as early as possible for any patient with complex medical needs.
- When collaborating with a subspecialist, communication is key. It is imperative from the beginning of the collaboration to the end to have effective, clear communication regarding the clinical question and treatment recommendations.
- The AAP recommends pediatric hospital medicine consultation if your patient is aged 14 years, more than 40 kg in weight, medically complex, or projected to exceed 24 LOS.[35]
- Pediatric ID consultation is recommended for patients with suspected or confirmed acute or chronic musculoskeletal infection in order to provide both acute intervention, establish a plan for disease surveillance and monitor for potential adverse effects of antibiotic therapy.
- There are specific evidence-based criteria regarding appropriate imaging for the diagnosis and screening of child physical abuse.[54] Both the AAP and the orthopedic literature provide guidelines to guide the medical evaluation in children whom physical abuse has been suspected.[32,55,56]
- Sentinel injuries (bruising to TEN-4 areas [Torso, Ear, Neck, <4 months of age]) are often a harbinger for other more serious injuries, and further screening for child abuse should be completed when these injuries are identified. To miss these injuries would put a child at risk for further injury or death.[29]
- The importance of documenting a thorough medical history that provides the necessary details regarding the mechanism of injury cannot be overstated. One study reported the pervasiveness of inadequate documentation of skeletal injuries in children and that there was poor indication in the medical record that abuse had been ruled out.[57]

DISCLOSURES

The authors have no disclosures.

REFERENCES

1. Baldwin DC Jr. Some historical notes on interdisciplinary and interprofessional education and practice in health care in the USA. 1996. J Interprof Care 2007;21(Suppl 1):23–37.
2. Rappaport DI, Adelizzi-Delany J, Rogers KJ, et al. Outcomes and costs associated with hospitalist comanagement of medically complex children undergoing spinal fusion surgery. Hosp Pediatr 2013;3(3):233–41.
3. The Joint Commission. Credentialing and Privileging-Consultants: Does the Joint Commission require licensed practitioners (LP) that provide consultative services to be credentialed or privileged? In: Critical Access Hospital-Joint Commission. 2016. Available at: https://www.jointcommission.org/standards/standard-faqs/hospital-and-hospital-clinics/medical-staff-ms/000002042/. Accessed October 14, 2022.
4. Dua K, McAvoy WC, Klaus SA, et al. Hospitalist comanagement of pediatric orthopaedic surgical patients at a community hospital. Md Med 2016;17(1):34–6.
5. SHM. Society of Hospital Medicine. Resources for effective co-management of hospitalized patients. Available at: https://www.hospitalmedicine.org/practice-management/co-management. Retrieved October 10, 2022.
6. Simon TD, Eilert R, Dickinson LM, et al. Pediatric hospitalist comanagement of spinal fusion surgery patients. J Hosp Med 2007;2(1):23–30.
7. Rohatgi N, Weng Y, Ahuja N. Surgical comanagement by hospitalists: continued improvement over 5 years. J Hosp Med 2020;15(4):232–5.
8. Rosenberg RE, Abzug JM, Rappaport DI, et al. Collaborations with pediatric hospitalists: National surveys of pediatric surgeons and orthopedic surgeons. J Hosp Med 2018;13(8):566–9.
9. Huddleston JM, Long KH, Naessens JM, et al. Medical and surgical comanagement after elective hip and knee arthroplasty: a randomized, controlled trial. Ann Intern Med 2004;141(1):28–38.
10. Taniguchi Y, Oichi T, Ohya J, et al. In-hospital mortality and morbidity of pediatric scoliosis surgery in Japan: Analysis using a national inpatient database. Medicine 2018;97(14):e0277.
11. Sullivan DJ, Primhak RA, Bevan C, et al. Complications in pediatric scoliosis surgery. Pediatr Anesth 2014;24:406–11.
12. Yuan N, Skaggs DL, Dorey F, et al. Preoperative predictors of prolonged postoperative mechanical ventilation in children following scoliosis repair. Pediatr Pulmonol 2005;40:414–9.
13. Moody C, Hayes S, Rusin N, et al. Risk assessment for postoperative pneumonia in children living with

neurologic impairments. Pediatrics 2021;148(3). e2021050130.
14. McQuivey KS, Chung AS, Jones MR, et al. Hospital outcomes in pediatric patients with Prader-Willi syndrome (PWS) undergoing orthopedic surgery: A 12-year analysis of national trends in surgical management and inpatient hospital outcomes [published online ahead of print, 2021]. J Orthop Sci 2021. https://doi.org/10.1016/j.jos.2021.08.005.
15. Jain A, Puvanesarajah V, Menga EN, et al. Unplanned hospital readmissions and reoperations after pediatric spinal fusion surgery. Spine 2015; 40(11):856–62.
16. Miller NH, Benefield E, Hastings L, et al. Evaluation of high-risk patients undergoing spinal surgery: a matched case series. J Pediatr Orthop 2010;30: 496–502.
17. Visser TG, Lehman EB, Armstron DG. Does routine subspecialty consultation before high-risk pediatric spine surgery decrease the incidence of complications? J Pediatr Orthop 2022;42(10):571–6.
18. Sheehan DD, Grayhack J. Pulmonary implications of pediatric spinal deformities. Pediatr Clin N Am 2021;68:239–59.
19. Prentice KM, Tsirikos AI, Urquhart DS. Pre-operative respiratory assessment for children with spinal deformity. Paediatr Respir Rev 2022;43:60–6.
20. Alsherhi A, Afshar K, Bedford J, et al. The relationship between preoperative nutritional state and adverse outcome following abdominal and thoracic surgery in children: Results from the NSQIP database. J Pediatr Surg 2018;53:1046–51.
21. Roberson ML, Egberg MD, Strassle PD, et al. Measuring malnutrition and its impact on pediatric surgery outcomes: a NSQIP-P analysis. J Pediatr Surg 2021;56:439–45.
22. Ladd MR, Garcia AV, Leeds IL, et al. Malnutrition increased the risk of 30-day complications after surgery in pediatric patients with Crohn disease. J Pediatr Surg 2018;53(11):2336–45.
23. Jevsevar DS, Karlin LI. The relationship between preoperative nutritional status and complications after and operation for scoliosis in patients who had cerebral palsy. J Bone Joint Surg 1993;75-A(6):880–4.
24. Martins DS, Piper HG. Nutrition considerations in pediatric surgical patients. Nutr Clin Pract 2022; 37:510–20.
25. Obana KK, Fan BB, Bennett JT, et al. Pre-operative nutrition assessments do not improve outcomes in cerebral palsy patients undergoing varus derotational osteotomy. Medicine 2021;100(47):e27776.
26. Kocher MS, Kasser JR. Orthopaedic aspects of child abuse. J Am Acad Orthop Surg 2000;8(1):10–20.
27. Hicks RA, Laskey AL, Harris TL, et al. Consultations in child abuse pediatrics. Clin Pediatr (Phila) 2020; 59(8):809–15.
28. Jenny C, Hymel KP, Ritzen A, et al. Analysis of missed cases of abusive head trauma [published correction appears in JAMA 1999 Jul 7;282(1):29]. JAMA 1999;281(7):621–6.
29. Block RW, Palusci VJ. Child abuse pediatrics: a new pediatric subspecialty. J Pediatr 2006;148(6):711–2.
30. McGuire L, Martin KD, Leventhal JM. Child abuse consultations initiated by child protective services: the role of expert opinions. Acad Pediatr 2011; 11(6):467–73.
31. Anderst J, Kellogg N, Jung I. Is the diagnosis of physical abuse changed when child protective services consults a child abuse pediatrics subspecialty group as a second opinion? Child Abuse Negl 2009;33(8):481–9.
32. Sink EL, Hyman JE, Matheny T, et al. Child abuse: the role of the orthopaedic surgeon in nonaccidental trauma. Clin Orthop Relat Res 2011;469(3):790–7.
33. Ranade SC, Allen AK, Deutsch SA. The role of the orthopaedic surgeon in the identification and management of nonaccidental trauma. J Am Acad Orthop Surg 2020;28(2):53–65.
34. Pacitti K, Mathew A, Royse A, et al. Hospitalist versus subspecialist perspectives on reasons, timing, and impact of consultation. J Healthc Qual 2017;39(6):367–78.
35. Rauch Daniel A, et al. Physician's role in coordinating care of hospitalized children. Pediatrics 2018;142(2):e20181503.
36. Anstey J, Lucas BP. Worry loves company, but unnecessary consultations may harm the patients we comanage. J Hosp Med 2020;15(1):60–1.
37. Siegal EM. Just because you can, doesn't mean that you should: a call for the rational application of hospitalist comanagement. J Hosp Med 2008; 3(5):398–402.
38. Rappaport DI, Pressel DM. Pediatric hospitalist comanagement of surgical patients: challenges and opportunities. Clin Pediatr (Phila) 2008;47(2): 114–21.
39. Gwee A, Carapetis JR, Buttery J, et al. Formal infectious diseases consultations at a tertiary pediatric hospital: a 14-year review. Pediatr Infect Dis J 2014;33(4):411–3.
40. Auzin A, Spits M, Tacconelli E, et al. What is the evidence base of used aggregated antibiotic resistance percentages to change empirical antibiotic treatment? a scoping review. Clin Microbiol Infect 2022;28(7):928–35.
41. Norris AH, Shrestha NK, Allison GM, et al. 2018 Infectious Diseases Society of America Clinical Practice Guideline for the Management of Outpatient Parenteral Antimicrobial Therapy. Clin Infect Dis 2019;68(1):e1–35.
42. Petrak RM, Sexton DJ, Butera ML, et al. The value of an infectious diseases specialist. Clin Infect Dis 2003;36(8):1013–7.

43. Jenkins TC, Price CS, Sabel AL, et al. Impact of routine infectious diseases service consultation on the evaluation, management, and outcomes of *Staphylococcus aureus* bacteremia. Clin Infect Dis 2008;46(7):1000–8.
44. Eron LJ, Passos S. Early discharge of infected patients through appropriate antibiotic use. Arch Intern Med 2001;161(1):61–5.
45. Gómez J, Conde Cavero SJ, Hernández Cardona JL, et al. The influence of the opinion of an infectious disease consultant on the appropriateness of antibiotic treatment in a general hospital. J Antimicrob Chemother 1996;38(2): 309–14.
46. Bork JT, Claeys KC, Heil EL, et al. A propensity score matched study of the positive impact of infectious diseases consultation on antimicrobial appropriateness in hospitalized patients with antimicrobial stewardship oversight. Antimicrob Agents Chemother 2020;64(8):e00307–20.
47. Fox BC, Imrey PB, Voights MB, et al. Infectious disease consultation and microbiologic surveillance for intensive care unit trauma patients: a pilot study. Clin Infect Dis 2001;33(12):1981–9.
48. Lahey T, Shah R, Gittzus J, et al. Infectious diseases consultation lowers mortality from *Staphylococcus aureus* bacteremia. Medicine (Baltim) 2009;88(5): 263–7.
49. Esposito S, Russo E, De Simone G, et al. Diagnostic and therapeutic appropriateness in bone and joint infections: results of a national survey. J Chemother 2016;28(3):191–7.
50. Schmitt S, McQuillen DP, Nahass R, et al. Infectious diseases specialty intervention is associated with decreased mortality and lower healthcare costs. Clin Infect Dis 2014;58(1):22–8.
51. Woods CR, Bradley JS, Chatterjee A, et al. Clinical practice guideline by the pediatric infectious diseases society and the infectious diseases society of America: 2021 guideline on diagnosis and management of acute hematogenous osteomyelitis in pediatrics. J Pediatric Infect Dis Soc 2021;10(8): 801–44.
52. Duguid RC, Al Reesi M, Bartlett AW, et al. Impact of infectious diseases consultation on management and outcome of Staphylococcus aureus bacteremia in children. J Pediatric Infect Dis Soc 2021;10(5): 569–75.
53. Mehler K, Oberthür A, Yagdiran A, et al. Impact of a pediatric infectious disease consultation service on timely step-down to oral antibiotic treatment for bone and joint infections. Infection 2022. https://doi.org/10.1007/s15010-022-01934-4.
54. Expert Panel on Pediatric Imaging, Wootton-Gorges SL, Soares BP, et al. ACR appropriateness criteria suspected physical abuse-child. J Am Coll Radiol 2017;14(5S):S338–49.
55. Jayakumar P, Barry M, Ramachandran M. Orthopaedic aspects of paediatric nonaccidental injury. J Bone Joint Surg Br 2010;92:189–95.
56. Sullivan CM. Child abuse and the legal system: The orthopaedic surgeon's role in diagnosis. Clin Orthop Relat Res 2011;469:768–75.
57. Oral R, Blum KL, Johnson C. Fractures in young children: are physicians in the emergency department and orthopedic clinics adequately screening for possible abuse? Pediatr Emerg Care 2003; 19(3):148–53.

Type 1 Diabetes Overview and Perioperative Management

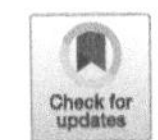

Grace B. Nelson, MD*, Kathryn M. Sumpter, MD

KEYWORDS

• Type 1 diabetes mellitus • Perioperative care • Surgery • Insulin infusion systems
• Hybrid closed-loop • Continuous glucose monitoring systems

KEY POINTS

- Treatment regimens for patients with type 1 diabetes (T1D) have become more variable and complex.
- Surgery can lead to increased glucose variability, which contributes to worse outcomes.
- Clear guidelines for blood sugar monitoring and insulin administration in the perioperative space provide improved patient care.
- Taking patients' current regimen into account is important for optimal care.

INTRODUCTION

Type 1 diabetes (T1D) is caused by the autoimmune destruction of the insulin-producing beta cells in the pancreatic islets of Langerhans.[1] It is the most common cause of diabetes among children and adolescents, and its incidence is increasing worldwide at an estimated rate of 2% to 4% per year.[2–5] Treatment regimens for patients with T1D have become more variable and complex with newer insulin analogues and increasing use of diabetes technology such as continuous subcutaneous insulin infusion, commonly referred to as insulin pumps, and continuous glucose monitoring (CGM) devices. Although current regimens provide increased flexibility for patients and improve both metabolic control and quality of life,[6,7] most of the pediatric and adult patients with T1D do not reach glycemic management targets.[8] With these more complicated treatment regimens and recognition of the risks of dysglycemia in the perioperative period, management of T1D in the surgical patient has become more complex as well. Careful planning and close monitoring are crucial to reducing the risks of dysglycemia and improving surgical outcomes for patients with T1D.

IMPACT OF ANESTHESIA AND SURGERY ON GLUCOSE METABOLISM

Both surgery and anesthesia are known to trigger a characteristic stress response that causes dramatic metabolic changes in the surgical patient with upregulation of counterregulatory hormone release and suppression of insulin secretion.[9–11] Counterregulatory hormones, which include cortisol, growth hormone, glucagon, epinephrine, and norepinephrine, promote catabolism, which includes glycogen release from the liver and gluconeogenesis, ultimately causing increased serum glucose. Insulin is the body's primary anabolic hormone, stimulating glycogen storage and peripheral glucose uptake in the skeletal muscle and adipose. By lowering insulin and increasing counterregulatory hormones, especially cortisol and catecholamines, surgery and anesthesia cause increased glucose release into the circulation with reduced glucose uptake in the periphery, potentially resulting in significant hyperglycemia and even

Pediatrics, University of Tennessee Health Science Center, 49 North Dunlap Street, Memphis, TN 38105, USA
* Corresponding author.
E-mail address: gbazan@uthsc.edu

Orthop Clin N Am 54 (2023) 287–298
https://doi.org/10.1016/j.ocl.2023.02.001
0030-5898/23/

diabetic ketoacidosis among patients with T1D.[12,13] The required preoperative nil per os status, reduction in preoperative insulin doses recommended in some cases, poor oral intake postoperatively due to nausea and/or pain, and continued stress response after surgery maintain and further amplify the catabolic response and resulting glycemic dysregulation.

RISKS OF DYSGLYCEMIA IN THE PERIOPERATIVE PERIOD

Hyperglycemia results in multiple adverse impacts in the perioperative patient. Elevated blood glucose leads to impaired neutrophil function including decreased chemotaxis, phagocytosis, and formation of reactive oxygen species,[14] which can increase the risk of perioperative infection. It is also associated with impaired healing of surgical wounds due to reduced production of collagen,[15] endothelial cell dysfunction[16] and disruption of migration, and proliferation of keratinocytes and fibroblasts.[17] Numerous studies have shown an association between perioperative glycemic control and risk of infection and other morbidities,[18–20] and interventions to improve glycemic control have reduced morbidity in several studies.[20,21]

Hypoglycemia also presents possible risks for the perioperative patient with T1D. Anesthesia may blunt the typical adrenergic symptoms of hypoglycemia and delay its recognition, increasing the risk of severe morbidity including irreversible neurologic damage.[22] Although initial studies suggested improved morbidity and mortality from "tight" glycemic control (ie, aiming for glucose between 80 and 110 mg/dL [4.5–6.1 mmol/L]) among critically ill patients,[21] later studies demonstrated considerable risk of this approach due to increased frequency of hypoglycemia.[23,24] Based on this, there is broad consensus behind aiming to maintain glucose less than 180 mg/dL (10 mmol/L) in the perioperative period, with some groups allowing an increase to 216 mg/dL (12 mmol/L) in selected cases. Although there is variability on the recommended target for the lower end of glucose, most guidelines recommend somewhere between 80 and 108 mg/dL (4.5–6.0 mmol/L).[25–27]

INSULIN ANALOGUES

Insulin analogues have changed significantly since the discovery of insulin in 1921.[28,29] There are now multiple types of insulin, with the most common types of insulin used in T1D being long-acting, rapid-acting, and ultra-rapid-acting (**Table 1**). Examples of long-acting insulin, also referred to as basal insulin, include glargine, degludec, and determir.[30] The goal of long-acting insulin is to keep blood sugar stable between meals and overnight.[29] Ideally a patient should be able to fast overnight without hypoglycemia or hyperglycemia after administration of long-acting insulin. Patients on insulin pumps typically do not take long-acting insulin injections and will require long-acting insulin administration if there is a plan to stop the insulin pump for a prolonged time perioperatively.[31] Ultra-rapid and rapid-acting insulins include aspart, lispro-aabc, faster aspart, lispro, and glulisine.[30] These insulins have an onset time of 5 to 15 minutes, peak action of 1 to 2 hours, and duration of action of 2 to 5 hours.[30] Ultra-rapid and rapid-acting insulin are used to correct hyperglycemia and cover the carbohydrates consumed in food. Most patients with T1D on multiple daily injection therapy take 1 to 2 injections of basal insulin daily and 3 or more injections of ultra-rapid- or rapid-acting insulin daily. Other types of insulin less commonly used for management of T1D include short-acting regular insulin and intermediate-acting Neutral Protamine Hagedorn insulin.[30] Regular insulin has a slower onset time of 30 minutes, with peak of 2 to 3 hours and duration of 6.5 hours when used subcutaneously, making it less useful for most situations of eating or correcting hyperglycemia.[30] Regular insulin is commonly used for intravenous (IV) administration of insulin.

INSULIN PUMPS AND CONTINUOUS GLUCOSE MONITORS

Insulin pumps have become more commonplace in the management of T1D. Insulin pumps use only rapid-acting insulin, which is given continuously to keep blood glucose steady between meals and overnight (ie, basal rate) and also as boluses for high blood sugar correction and when eating carbs. Current data suggest that approximately 50% of patients in the United States with T1D use insulin pumps.[32] Insulin pumps have a subcutaneous needle or cannula that is inserted by the patient and must be replaced every 2 to 3 days. There are broadly 2 types of pumps, those with tubing and those without (**Fig. 1**). For tubeless pumps, the insulin reservoir and insertion site are contained within a "pod" that adheres directly to the skin at the insertion site. For pumps with tubing, the insertion site is connected via tubing to a reservoir that sits within a small device that can then be placed in a pocket or clipped to clothing.

Table 1
Insulin analogues: differences and uses

Insulin Name	Onset Time	Peak Time	Duration of Action	Common Outpatient Use	Common Inpatient Use
Very rapid-acting insulin					
Fast-aspart	4 min	1–2 h	3–5 h	Mealtime and high blood sugar correction	For meals and corrections, ok to sub aspart or lispro
Lispro-aabc	2 min	1–2 h	4.6 h	Mealtime and high blood sugar correction	Usually not on formularies, ok to sub aspart or lispro
Rapid-Acting insulin: generally ok to substitute any of the rapid-acting insulins based on formulary					
Aspart	10–15 min	1–3 h	3–5 h	Insulin pump, mealtime and high blood sugar correction	Insulin pump, mealtime and high blood sugar correction
Glulisine	10–15 min	1–2 h	2–4 h	Insulin pump, mealtime and high blood sugar correction	Insulin pump, mealtime and high blood sugar correction
Lispro	10–15 min	1–2 h	3–5 h	Insulin pump, mealtime and high blood sugar correction	Insulin pump, mealtime and high blood sugar correction
Short-acting insulin					
Regular	30 min	2–3h	6.5 h	Not typically used outpatient	Used in IV drips of insulin
Intermediate-acting insulin					
NPH	1–3 h	5–8 h	18 h	In mixed insulins	Not typically used
Detemir	3–4 h	6–8 h	18 h	1–2x daily basal insulin	Should be continued inpatient, ok to sub glargine if detemir not on formulary
Long-acting insulin					
Glargine	1.5 h	No peak	24 h	Once daily basal insulin	Should be continued inpatient
Degludec	30–90 min	No peak	42 h	Once daily basal insulin	Should be continued inpatient, ok to sub glargine if degludec not on formulary

Abbreviation: NPH, Neutral Protamine Hagedorn.

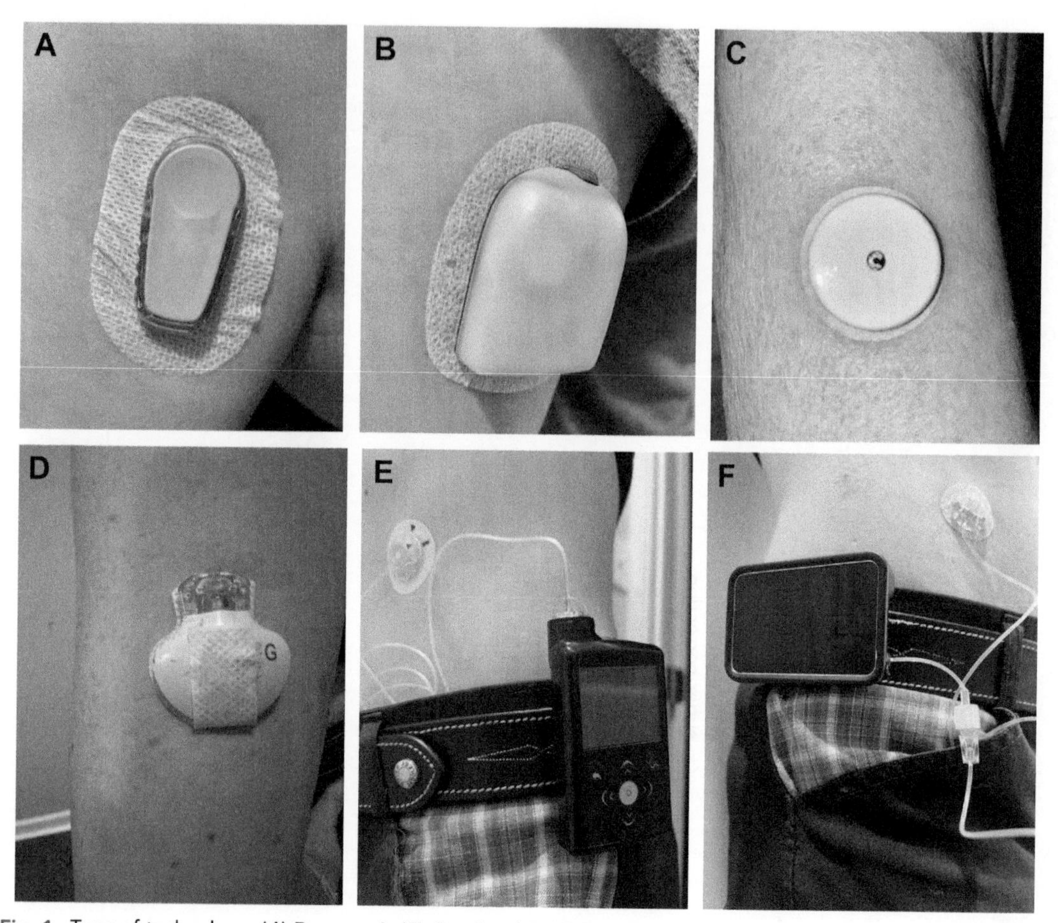

Fig. 1. Type of technology. (*A*) Dexcom 6, (*B*) Omnipod 5, (*C*) FreeStyle Libre (*D*), Medtronic Guardian CGM, (*E*) Medtronic 670G pump, and (*F*) Tandem Tslim X2 pump.

Although insulin pumps with tubing can be disconnected from the insertion site and reconnected without starting a whole new "set," tubeless pumps cannot be removed and then replaced without using a new "pod." For surgeries less than 3 hours long, it may be safe to leave an insulin pump in place.[31] Pumps must be removed for MRI or computed tomography (CT), although a lead shield may be sufficient for radiographs based on the manufacturer's recommendation.[31] If the pump is removed for longer than 1 hour, the patient must be given an alternate insulin source to prevent hyperglycemia and ketosis.

CGM have rapidly become standard of care for patients with T1D over the last 10 years. Currently approximately 50% of patients with T1D in the United States use CGM.[33] CGM are small devices that monitor glucose continuously by sensing the interstitial fluid glucose concentrations every 5 minutes (see Fig. 1). As a consequence of the COVID-19 pandemic, there has been an increase in use of CGM in the inpatient setting, as hospitals sought to limit staff exposure to the virus while maintaining adequate glycemic monitoring.[34,35] Although CGMs are not yet Food and Drug Administration (FDA)-approved for inpatient use, the FDA is now exercising enforcement discretion for the use of these factory-calibrated devices in the hospital setting, both to facilitate patient care and to obtain performance data to be used for further regulatory submission.[34] With appropriate policies and procedures in place, CGMs can be used to decrease frequency of fingersticks for point-of-care capillary blood glucose testing while also decreasing glucose variability and preventing severe hypoglycemia.[34,35] One important caveat of using any CGM in the hospital is that they are not cleared for use in MRI, CT, or radiography (Table 2) and thus would need to be removed for imaging, which could prove wasteful, as once a CGM sensor is removed a new one must be placed.[35] One study used simulated radiation and magnetic exposure to demonstrate no change in dextrose sensing

Table 2
Continuous glucose monitoring systems, interfering substances and radiation tolerance

Device	Interfering Substances	Radiation Tolerance
Dexcom G6	Hydroxyurea	No clinical studies. Radiograph may be ok. Remove for CT, MRI, or heat therapy
Freestyle libre 2	Ascorbic acid	No clinical studies. Radiograph may be ok. Remove for CT, MRI, or heat therapy
Freestyle libre	Ascorbic acid Salicylic acid	No clinical studies. Radiograph may be ok. Remove for CT, MRI, or heat therapy
Medtronic guardian sensor 3	Acetaminophen	No clinical studies. Radiograph may be ok. Remove for CT, MRI, or heat therapy
Senseonics eversense	Mannitol tetracycline	Nonclinical studies show MRI may be fine. Radiograph and CT are fine

From Galindo RJ et al. Continuous Glucose Monitors and Automated Insulin Dosing Systems in the Hospital Consensus Guideline. J Diabetes Sci Technol. 2020 Nov;14(6):1035-1064. https://doi.org/10.1177/1932296820954163. Epub 2020 Sep 28. PMID: 32985262; PMCID: PMC7645140.

ability of the Dexcom G6.[36] Some sites have covered the CGM device with a lead shield, and no adverse events have yet been reported with this practice.[35]

The newest technological advance for T1D care is the hybrid closed-loop (HCL) system, also known as automated insulin delivery system. These systems integrate CGMs with insulin pumps using an algorithm to adjust insulin delivery based on current glucose level and trends from the CGM.[35] HCL systems have greatly improved quality of life and eased burden of diabetes management for many patients, and many patients prefer to stay on these systems when admitted to the hospital.[35] Although hospitals may have different policies for use of CGM and insulin pumps, it is within the FDA's authorized use guidelines for a patient to use their own device for self-management while in the hospital.[35]

PREOPERATIVE PLANNING AND EVALUATION OF PATIENTS WITH TYPE 1 DIABETES

Thorough preoperative evaluation and planning are recommended to reduce perioperative risks for patients with T1D. First, one must assess the effectiveness of the patient's baseline diabetes management and feasibility of using their home regimen perioperatively. Although measures such as the CGM time in range and time above range are now widely used as important adjuncts for assessment of glycemic management and as a basis for clinical decision-making, hemoglobin A1c remains the standard metric for glycemic control.[37] Multiple studies demonstrate an association between higher baseline A1c and perioperative and postoperative complications.[38–40] Some argue this is simply because a higher baseline A1c is associated with higher perioperative glucose levels, but one study showed that a higher baseline A1c and higher perioperative glucose levels were independently associated with postoperative complications among patients undergoing emergency surgery and that having both conferred a 4-fold increased risk of complications.[41] Based on these data, it is clear that an A1c in the target range of less than 7%[37] would be optimal, but it is less clear how to approach cases in which A1c is greater than target. Some guidelines specify that elective surgeries should be delayed for patients with A1c greater than 8% to 9%,[31,42] whereas some centers require even lower targets. Data suggest it takes many patients longer than 6 months to lower A1c less than these targets and is not accomplished in others.[43] For patients with preoperative hemoglobin A1c greater than 8%, it is recommended that the surgeon, primary care provider, and endocrinologist collaborate to weigh the risks and benefits of proceeding with surgery versus delaying with the hope of improving baseline glycemic control. In cases where baseline glycemic control is poor but delaying surgery confers unacceptable risk, some institutions prefer inpatient admission for continuous IV insulin infusion the night before surgery to maintain glucose in the target range.

Next, the patient's baseline insulin regimen should be determined and recorded. For patients using multiple daily insulin injections, it is important to know the doses for long-acting insulin as well as the manner of dosing rapid-acting insulin. Some patients use a "sliding scale" at meals that includes a set dose of insulin for carbohydrates consumed along with a variable correction amount based on premeal glucose level, whereas other patients calculate insulin doses using an insulin-to-carbohydrate ratio and a correction factor. For patients using an insulin pump (with or without HCL technology), the pump is programmed with insulin-to-carbohydrate ratios and correction factors. The authors recommend documenting these values to allow insulin dosing in case of pump failure.

Consultation with the patient's diabetes care provider and close communication between that provider and the surgical team are both crucial to successful preoperative planning for patients with T1D; this is especially true for patients using intermediate-acting or mixed insulins where the regimen may need to be adjusted significantly leading up to surgery. For patients taking long-acting insulin (eg, glargine, detemir), some practitioners choose to lower the final dose given before surgery by 10% to 20% to lower the risk of hypoglycemia, whereas others feel strongly that the full baseline dose should be given to prevent hyperglycemia and ketosis. Similarly, some practitioners lower basal rates on an insulin pump by 10% to 20% during the hours of fasting before surgery, whereas others maintain basal rates without adjustment. Although one study among patients with type 2 diabetes demonstrated that a modest reduction in the basal insulin dose before surgery reduced the risk of hypoglycemia and increased the chance of arriving with glucose in target range on the day of surgery,[44] there are no evidence-based recommendations to guide these decisions for patients with T1D. The authors recommend they be made by the primary diabetes care provider based on their knowledge of the patient's baseline diabetes management and in consultation with the patient.

The time of day for surgery is important for a patient with T1D, as it will affect the duration of fasting. Longer fasting can increase the risk of hypoglycemia, so there is consensus that elective surgeries for patients with T1D should be scheduled as the first case of the day.[45–47]

Because the duration of surgery will affect the method chosen for intraoperative glucose control as well as the feasibility of continuing to use an insulin pump intraoperatively, it is critical to estimate the duration of the planned procedure. Available data and published experience suggest that insulin pumps may be safely used for procedures planned to be 2 hours or less, assuming it is permitted by institutional policy and the patient agrees.[46] For cases expected to last more than 3 hours, a variable rate IV insulin infusion (ie, insulin drip) allows for finer titration of glucose levels, whereas most shorter procedures can be managed with subcutaneous insulin via injections or a pump.

For patients using insulin pumps and/or CGMs, presurgical planning must consider whether the procedure will include radiography, CT, or MRI, as doing so may necessitate removal of the pump or CGM (see earlier section on "Insulin Pumps and Continuous Glucose Monitors").

If a patient will continue using their insulin pump during surgery, it is crucial that they arrive to surgery with the pump working properly. It is recommended that patients replace their infusion site or "pod" 12 to 24 hours before surgery to ensure the site is fresh, which leads to more consistent absorption compared with a site that has been present for more than 3 days.[48] Changing it at least 12 hours in advance also allows enough time to confirm that insulin is infusing well and the subcutaneous cannula is not kinked. Patients should be counseled to place the infusion site in a location that will be accessible to operating room staff but is outside the surgical field and will not be compressed by the patient's own body weight during the procedure. Similarly, for patients using HCL pumps during surgery, the CGM sensor must be placed in a location that is outside the surgical field and will not be compressed by the patient's own body weight during the procedure. In addition, the patient must ensure that CGM sensor will expire at least 24 hours after the planned procedure. If the sensor needs to be replaced, patients should do so 12 to 24 hours before surgery to ensure it has time to warm up and is working properly before the procedure.

DAY OF SURGERY MANAGEMENT

All patients should have point-of-care capillary blood glucose (BG) tested on arrival. If initial BG is less than 70 mg/dL (3.9 mmol/L), a 2 mL/kg IV bolus of 10% dextrose should be given and BG checked again in 15 minutes. Dextrose boluses can be repeated every 15 minutes until BG is greater than 70 mg/dL. If initial BG is greater than 250 mg/dL (13.9 mmol/L), urine ketones should be checked. If urine ketones are moderate (30 mg/dL or 3 mmol/L) or greater, endocrinology should be consulted and surgery postponed until hyperglycemia and ketosis have improved. Typical perioperative care can continue if initial BG is between 70 and 250 mg/dL (3.9–13.9 mmol/L). See Figs. 1–3 for greater detail on recommendations based on initial BG.

For all procedures planned to last more than 3 hours, the authors recommend pausing the home insulin regimen and starting a variable rate IV insulin infusion at 0.01 to 0.02 units/kg/h (see Fig. 1). BG should be checked every hour, and insulin rate can be titrated to maintain glucose between 100 and 180 mg/dL (5.6–10 mmol/L). Fluids containing 5% dextrose at maintenance rate help maintain adequate hydration and prevent both ketosis and hypoglycemia.

Multiple Daily Injections

Patients using multiple daily injections can continue to receive subcutaneous insulin

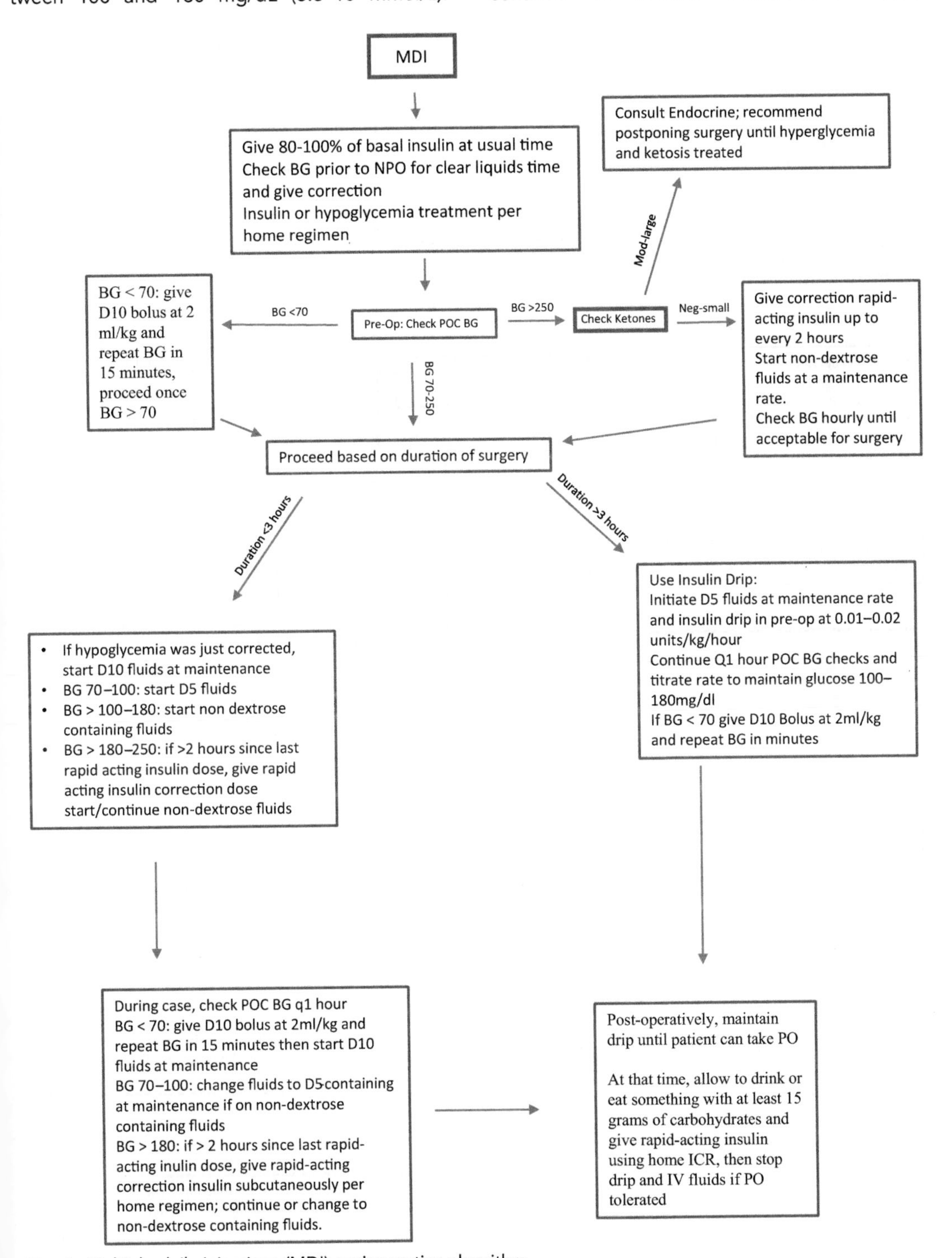

Fig. 2. Multiple daily injections (MDI) perioperative algorithm.

injections for perioperative diabetes management if the procedure will last less than 3 hours. After the initial BG check, IV fluids are started to maintain euvolemia and euglycemia. Dextrose content will vary based on initial BG level as outlined in Fig. 1. BG should be checked every hour during surgery with the goal of maintaining BG 100 to 180 mg/dL (5.6–10 mmol/L). If BG is less than 100 mg/dL (5.6 mmol/L) or greater than 180 mg/dL (10 mmol/L), see Fig. 1 for recommendations on adjusting fluids and giving supplemental rapid-acting insulin based on the BG level.

Postoperatively, IV fluids can be stopped once the patient is able to eat or drink at least

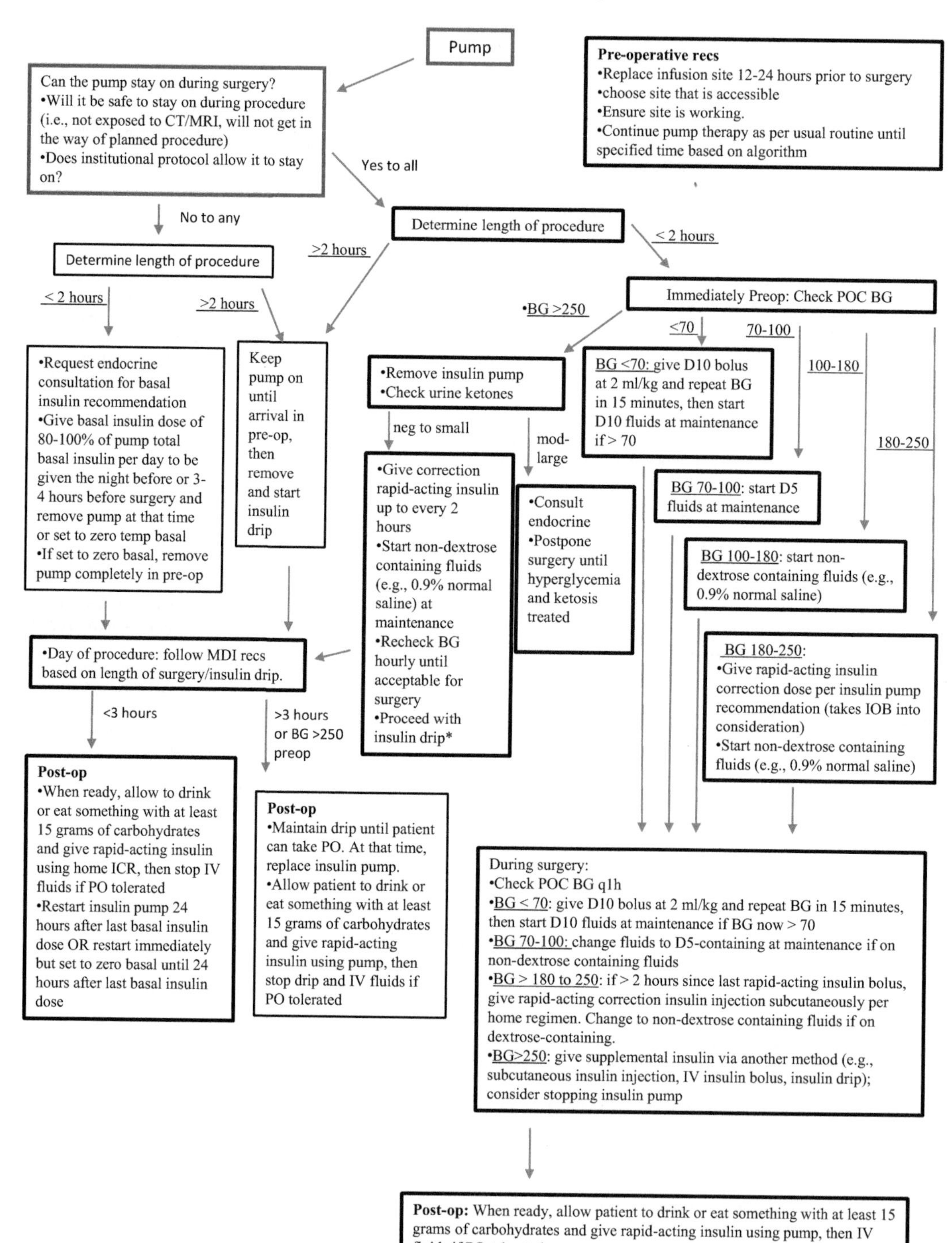

Fig. 3. Pump perioperative algorithm.

15 g of carbohydrates. Rapid-acting insulin should be given for the carbohydrates consumed using the patient's home insulin-to-carbohydrate ratio.

Insulin Pump

Patients using their open-loop insulin pump during surgery will be started on IV fluids after initial BG check to maintain euvolemia and euglycemia. Dextrose content will vary based on initial BG level as outlined in Fig. 2. If preoperative BG is between 180 and 250 mg/dL (10–13.9 mmol/L), supplemental insulin may be given using the insulin pump bolus calculator (see Fig. 2), which adjusts the recommended bolus based on "insulin on board," which is an estimation of the insulin still active in the body from boluses given over the last several hours. If initial BG is greater than 250 mg/dL (10–13.9 mmol/L), urine ketones should be checked as outlined earlier, and the insulin pump should be removed and not used during surgery. If the insulin pump

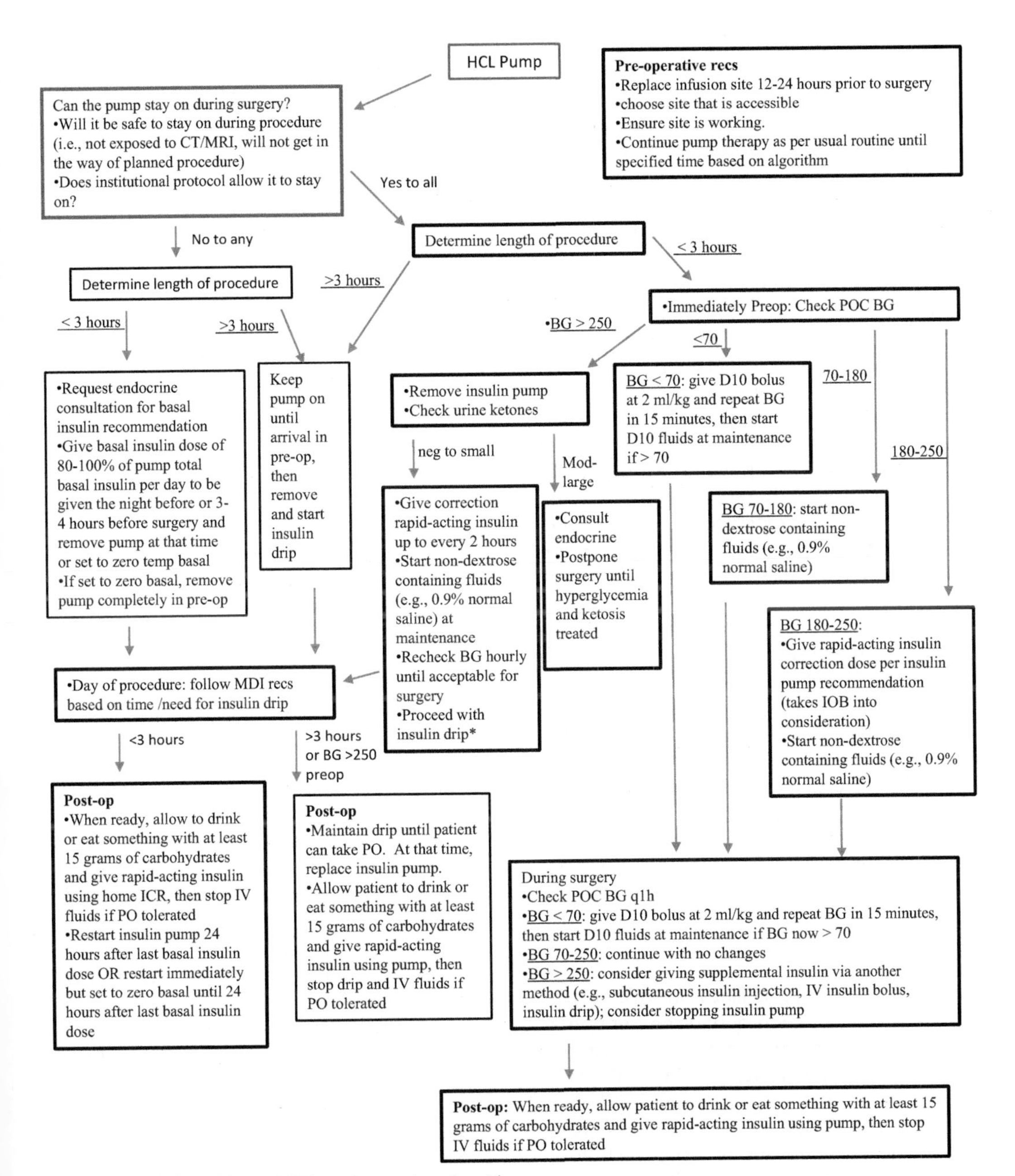

Fig. 4. Hybrid closed-loop (HCL) perioperative algorithm.

is removed, an alternate insulin source must be provided, as patients using insulin pumps do not take basal insulin to prevent worsening of hyperglycemia and ketosis. The authors recommend using a variable rate IV insulin infusion during the procedure as described earlier and restarting the insulin pump postoperatively.

For patients continuing to use their insulin pump during surgery, intraoperative BG should be checked every hour with the goal of maintaining BG 100 to 180 mg/dL (5.6–10 mmol/L). Fig. 2 outlines recommendations on adjusting fluids and giving supplemental, subcutaneous rapid-acting insulin if BG is less than100 mg/dL (5.6 mmol/L) or greater than 180 mg/dL (10 mmol/L).

Postoperatively, IV fluids can be stopped once the patient is able to eat or drink at least 15 g of carbohydrates. Rapid-acting insulin should be given through the insulin pump for the carbohydrates consumed via a bolus programmed by the patient or guardian.

Hybrid Closed-Loop Insulin Pump

Perioperative management for patients using an HCL insulin pump during surgery is very similar to using an open-loop insulin pump but there are some differences (Fig. 3). First, giving dextrose-containing fluids during the procedure is not necessary for most patients, as the system adjusts insulin delivery to reduce the risk of both hyperglycemia and hypoglycemia. Also, giving subcutaneous insulin injections during the procedure for BG less than 250 mg/dL (13.9 mmol/L) is not recommended, as the HCL system increases insulin delivery for hyperglycemia, and giving an insulin injection in addition to the pump's insulin delivery could cause hypoglycemia.

As is the case for open-loop pumps, IV fluids can be stopped postoperatively once the patient using HCL is able to eat or drink at least 15 g of carbohydrates. Rapid-acting insulin should be given through the HCL pump for the carbohydrates consumed via a bolus programmed by the patient or guardian (Fig. 4).

SUMMARY

T1D is a complex, chronic illness in which glycemic variability is common during the perioperative period and for which management can be challenging. Recent advances in T1D care, including newer insulin analogues and technologies such as CGMs and HCL pumps, have improved quality of life and reduced the burden of care for patients with T1D while also increasing the complexity of perioperative management for such patients. With adequate preoperative planning and intraoperative monitoring, these devices can be used successfully during many surgical cases. For all patients with T1D undergoing surgery, the surgical team must carefully assess the patient's surgical risk, determine the most appropriate plan for perioperative diabetes management in consultation with the patient and their primary diabetes care provider, and ensure assiduous monitoring of blood glucose levels and consistent adherence to the perioperative diabetes management plan throughout. Doing so will reduce the risks of surgery-associated dysglycemia and may improve surgical outcomes for patients with T1D.

CLINICS CARE POINTS

- Determine baseline diabetes care regimen and blood glucose targets.
- Attempt to continue home regimens as much as possible when appropriate.
- Discuss plans with Diabetes Care provider.
- Recognize need for adjustments based glucose levels at time of surgery.

DISCLOSURE

The authors have nothing to disclose.

REFERENCES

1. Eisenbarth GS. Type I diabetes mellitus: a chronic autoimmune disease. N Engl J Med 1986;314(21):1360–8.
2. Group DP. Incidence and trends of childhood type 1 diabetes worldwide 1990-1999. Diabet Med 2006;23(8):857–66.
3. Vehik K, Hamman RF, Lezotte D, et al. Increasing incidence of type 1 diabetes in 0- to 17-year-old Colorado youth. Diabetes Care 2007;30(3):503–9.
4. Patterson CC.
5. Lawrence JM, Divers J, Isom S, et al. Trends in prevalence of type 1 and type 2 diabetes in children and adolescents in the US, 2001-2017. JAMA 2021;326(8):717–27.
6. Cherubini V, Gesuita R, Bonfanti R, et al. Health-related quality of life and treatment preferences in adolescents with type 1 diabetes. The VIPKIDS study. Acta Diabetol 2014;51(1):43–51.
7. Hussain T, Akle M, Nagelkerke N, et al. Comparative study on treatment satisfaction and health

perception in children and adolescents with type 1 diabetes mellitus on multiple daily injection of insulin, insulin pump and sensor-augmented pump therapy. SAGE Open Med 2017;5. 2050312117694938.
8. Foster NC, Beck RW, Miller KM, et al. State of type 1 diabetes management and outcomes from the T1D exchange in 2016-2018. Diabetes Technol Ther 2019;21(2):66–72.
9. Allison SP, Tomlin PJ, Chamberlain MJ. Some effects of anaesthesia and surgery on carbohydrate and fat metabolism. Br J Anaesth 1969;41(7): 588–93.
10. Halter JB, Pflug AE. Relationship of impaired insulin secretion during surgical stress to anesthesia and catecholamine release. J Clin Endocrinol Metab 1980;51(5):1093–8.
11. Desborough JP. The stress response to trauma and surgery. Br J Anaesth 2000;85(1):109–17.
12. Schricker T, Lattermann R. Perioperative catabolism. Can J Anaesth 2015;62(2):182–93.
13. Hirsch IB, McGill JB. Role of insulin in management of surgical patients with diabetes mellitus. Diabetes Care 1990;13(9):980–91.
14. Turina M, Fry DE, Polk HC Jr. Acute hyperglycemia and the innate immune system: clinical, cellular, and molecular aspects. Crit Care Med 2005;33(7): 1624–33.
15. Rosenberg CS. Wound healing in the patient with diabetes mellitus. Nurs Clin North Am 1990;25(1): 247–61.
16. Koitka A, Abraham P, Bouhanick B, et al. Impaired pressure-induced vasodilation at the foot in young adults with type 1 diabetes. Diabetes 2004;53(3): 721–5.
17. Burgess JL, Wyant WA, Abdo Abujamra B, et al. Diabetic Wound-Healing Science. Medicina (Kaunas) 2021;(10):57. https://doi.org/10.3390/medicina57101072.
18. Ramos M, Khalpey Z, Lipsitz S, et al. Relationship of perioperative hyperglycemia and postoperative infections in patients who undergo general and vascular surgery. Ann Surg 2008;248(4):585–91.
19. Sathya B, Davis R, Taveira T, et al. Intensity of perioperative glycemic control and postoperative outcomes in patients with diabetes: a meta-analysis. Diabetes Res Clin Pract 2013;102(1):8–15.
20. Furnary AP, Zerr KJ, Grunkemeier GL, et al. Continuous intravenous insulin infusion reduces the incidence of deep sternal wound infection in diabetic patients after cardiac surgical procedures. Ann Thorac Surg 1999;67(2):352–60. ; discussion 360-2.
21. van den Berghe G, Wouters P, Weekers F, et al. Intensive insulin therapy in critically ill patients. N Engl J Med 2001;345(19):1359–67.
22. Kalra S, Bajwa SJ, Baruah M, et al. Hypoglycaemia in anesthesiology practice: diagnostic, preventive, and management strategies. Saudi J Anaesth 2013;7(4):447–52.
23. Investigators N-SS, Finfer S, Chittock DR, et al. Intensive versus conventional glucose control in critically ill patients. N Engl J Med 2009;360(13): 1283–97.
24. Preiser JC, Devos P, Ruiz-Santana S, et al. A prospective randomised multi-centre controlled trial on tight glucose control by intensive insulin therapy in adult intensive care units: the Glucontrol study. Intensive Care Med 2009;35(10):1738–48.
25. Guideline for Perioperative Care for People with Diabetes Mellitus Undergoing Elective and Emergency Surgery. Centre for Perioperative Care (CPOC); Available at: https://www.cpoc.org.uk/sites/cpoc/files/documents/2021-03/CPOC-Guideline%20for%20Perioperative%20Care%20for%20People%20with%20Diabetes%20Mellitus%20Undergoing%20Elective%20and%20Emergency%20Surgery.pdf; 2021.
26. American Diabetes Association Professional Practice Committee, American Diabetes Association Professional Practice Committee, Draznin B., et al., 16. Diabetes care in the hospital: standards of medical care in diabetes-2022, *Diabetes Care*, **45** (Suppl 1), 2022, S244–S253. doi: 10.2337/dc22-S016. PMID: 34964884.
27. Cheisson G, Jacqueminet S, Cosson E, et al. Perioperative management of adult diabetic patients. Intraoperative period. Anaesth Crit Care Pain Med 2018;37(Suppl 1):S21–5.
28. Recmmendations Ped Anesth. 2021;doi:10.1213/ANE.0000000000004491.
29. Rodbard HW, Rodbard D. Biosynthetic human insulin and insulin analogs. Am J Ther 2020;27(1): e42–51.
30. Lee SH, Yoon KH. A century of progress in diabetes care with insulin: a history of innovations and foundation for the future. Diabetes Metab J 2021;45(5): 629–40.
31. Akiboye F, Rayman G. Management of hyperglycemia and diabetes in orthopedic surgery. Curr Diab Rep 2017;17(2):13.
32. Lyons SK, Ebekozien O, Garrity A, et al. Increasing insulin pump use among 12- to 26-year-olds with type 1 diabetes: results from the T1D exchange quality improvement collaborative. Clin Diabetes 2021;39(3):272–7.
33. DeSalvo DJ, Noor N, Xie C, et al. Patient demographics and clinical outcomes among type 1 diabetes patients using continuous glucose monitors: data from t1d exchange real-world observational study. J Diabetes Sci Technol 2021. https://doi.org/10.1177/19322968211049783. 19322968211049783.
34. Perez-Guzman MC, SDeSalvo DJ, Noor N, Xie C, et al. Continuous glucose monitoring in the type 1

diabetes overview and perioperative management 297 hospital. Endocrinol Metab (Seoul) 2021;36(2): 240–55. https://doi.org/10.3803/EnM.2021.201.
35. Galindo RJ, Umpierrez GE, Rushakoff RJ, et al. Continuous glucose monitors and automated insulin dosing systems in the hospital consensus guideline. J Diabetes Sci Technol 2020;14(6):1035–64.
36. Thomas C, Welsh JB, Lu S, et al. Safety and functional integrity of continuous glucose monitoring components after simulated radiologic procedures. J Diabetes Sci Technol 2021;15(4):781–5.
37. American Diabetes Association Professional Practice C, Draznin B, Aroda VR, et al. 6. Glycemic targets: standards of medical care in diabetes-2022. Diabetes Care 2022;45(Suppl 1):S83–96.
38. Underwood P, Askari R, Hurwitz S, et al. Preoperative A1C and clinical outcomes in patients with diabetes undergoing major noncardiac surgical procedures. Diabetes Care 2014;37(3):611–6.
39. Yong PH, Weinberg L, Torkamani N, et al. The presence of diabetes and higher HbA1c are independently associated with adverse outcomes after surgery. Diabetes Care 2018;41(6):1172–9.
40. Halkos ME, Puskas JD, Lattouf OM, et al. Elevated preoperative hemoglobin A1c level is predictive of adverse events after coronary artery bypass surgery. J Thorac Cardiovasc Surg 2008;136(3):631–40.
41. Jehan F, Khan M, Sakran JV, et al. Perioperative glycemic control and postoperative complications in patients undergoing emergency general surgery: What is the role of Plasma Hemoglobin A1c? J Trauma Acute Care Surg 2018;84(1):112–7.
42. Dhatariya K, Levy N, Kilvert A, et al. NHS Diabetes guideline for the perioperative management of the adult patient with diabetes. Diabet Med 2012;29(4): 420–33.
43. Giori NJ, Ellerbe LS, Bowe T, et al. Many diabetic total joint arthroplasty candidates are unable to achieve a preoperative hemoglobin A1c goal of 7% or less. J Bone Joint Surg Am 2014;96(6):500–4.
44. Demma LJ, Carlson KT, Duggan EW, et al. Effect of basal insulin dosage on blood glucose concentration in ambulatory surgery patients with type 2 diabetes. J Clin Anesth 2017;36:184–8.
45. Martin LD, Hoagland MA, Rhodes ET, et al. Perioperative management of pediatric patients with type 1 diabetes mellitus, updated recommendations for anesthesiologists. Anesth Analg 2020;130(4):821–7.
46. Partridge H, Perkins B, Mathieu S, et al. Clinical recommendations in the management of the patient with type 1 diabetes on insulin pump therapy in the perioperative period: a primer for the anaesthetist. Br J Anaesth 2016;116(1):18–26.
47. Simha V, Shah P. Perioperative glucose control in patients with diabetes undergoing elective surgery. JAMA 2019;321(4):399–400.
48. Swan KL, Dziura JD, Steil GM, et al. Effect of age of infusion site and type of rapid-acting analog on pharmacodynamic parameters of insulin boluses in youth with type 1 diabetes receiving insulin pump therapy. Diabetes Care 2009;32(2):240–4.

Hand and Wrist

Management of Gout in the Hand and Wrist

Hayden S. Holbrook, MD*, James H. Calandruccio, MD

KEYWORDS

• Gout • Hand • Wrist • Inflammatory arthritis • Hyperuricemia • Uric acid • Surgical treatment

KEY POINTS

- Gout, or monosodium urate deposition disease, is the most common form of inflammatory arthritis which affects almost 4% of adults in the United States.
- Medical management involves lifestyle modifications and urate lowering therapy to reduce the frequency of gout flares, decrease the tophi size, and improve upper extremity function.
- Goals for surgical management of gout include functional optimization, symptomatic treatment, and cosmetic restoration.
- This article focuses on the medical and surgical treatment for the common manifestations of gout in the upper extremity including tophi, tenosynovitis, joint contractures, neural compression, and arthropathy.

INTRODUCTION

Gout is the most common form of inflammatory arthritis in the world affecting 1% to 2% of the adult male population.[1] Epidemiologic studies have reported an increase in the prevalence and incidence of gout possibly due to changes in diet, alcohol consumption, and use of diuretic agents.[2] Most recently, data from the Center for Disease Control's National Health and Nutrition Examination Survey reported the prevalence of gout to be 3.9% in US adults in the year of 2015 to 2016.[3] This rate correlates with 9.2 million adults suffering from gout, up from 8.3 million patients a decade earlier. Gout is rare in premenopausal women, as they are protected by the uricosuric effect of estrogen.[4] Although gout is most prevalent in the first metatarsophalangeal joint, termed "podagra," urate deposition has been identified in 17% of hands of patients with gout.[5] Gouty tophi of the hand and wrist are common reasons why patients may seek the care of an upper extremity surgeon.

CAUSE: HYPERURICEMIA AND GOUT

Human plasma urate originates exogenously from foods containing purines and from endogenous purine synthesis. The definition of hyperuricemia varies but common definitions include serum urate levels greater than 2 standard deviations more than the mean or serum urate levels greater than 6.8 mg/dL, which is the concentration at which urate crystals form at physiologic pH and temperature.[6]

Hyperuricemia, and ultimately gout, is caused by either underexcretion or overproduction of uric acid. Two-thirds of urate excretion occurs through the kidneys and the remaining through the intestinal tract. Renal underexcretion is the dominant cause of gout that can be due to genetics, drug effects, toxins, or chronic kidney disease.[7,8] Antiuricosuric medications such as diuretics, levodopa, cyclosporine, tacrolimus, and ethambutol reduce renal uric acid excretion. Overproduction of uric acid accounts for only a minority of cases of gout occurring with chemotherapy treatment, hemolytic anemias, or hemoglobinopathies.

Campbell Clinic Department of Orthopaedic Surgery and Biomedical Engineering, University of Tennessee Health Science Center, Memphis, TN, USA
* Corresponding author. 1211 Union Avenue, Suite 500, Memphis, TN 38104.
E-mail address: hholbro2@uthsc.edu

Orthop Clin N Am 54 (2023) 299–308
https://doi.org/10.1016/j.ocl.2023.02.003
0030-5898/23/

Hyperuricemia
(without Crystals)
Hyperuricemia
with Crystals
Intermittent
Acute Gout
Flares
Chronic Gout
with structural
changes

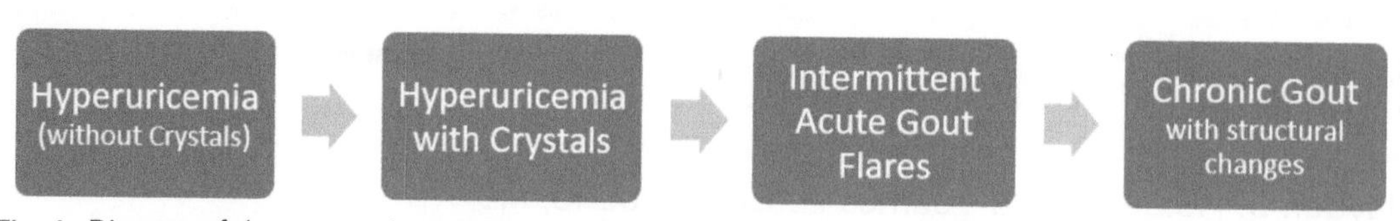

Fig. 1. Diagram of the temporal progression of gout due to long-standing hyperuricemia beginning with subclinical inflammation and ultimately leading to structural damage found in chronic gout.

Hyperuricemia and gout progress through 4 stages: (1) hyperuricemia without evidence of monosodium urate crystal deposition or gout, (2) crystal deposition without symptomatic gout, (3) crystal deposition with acute gout flares, and (4) advanced gout characterized by tophi, chronic gouty arthritis, and radiographic erosions (Fig. 1).[6] Gout occurs when persistent hyperuricemia causes monosodium urate crystal deposition. Crystal formation depends on a number of factors including temperature, pH, salt concentration, level of articular dehydration, and the presence of nucleating agents that most frequently align within peripheral joints to initiate crystallization.[6] These crystals initiate an inflammatory response mediated by the NLRP3 inflammasome within macrophages during an acute gout flare. In the chronic setting, this inflammatory process leads to gouty arthritis, erosions, and tophi in addition to various soft-tissue manifestations. Based on the evidence of several studies, the risk of gout flares and gouty arthritis is reduced at lower serum urate levels, which serves as the basis for the recommendation of urate-lowering therapy in patients with gout.[9–11]

LABORATORY EVALUATION

The gold standard for the diagnosis of gout is the presence of monosodium urate crystals on aspirated synovial fluid or from excised tophi. Gout crystals are needle shaped and negatively birefringent under polarizing light microscopy. Crystals can be identified by joint arthrocentesis during an acute flare as well as during the asymptomatic intercritical phase.[12] It is important to note that urate crystals are soluble in water and formalin, and if a tophi tissue sample is sent to the pathology laboratory in an aqueous solution, the urate will dissolve and crystals will not be found. For this reason, the sample should be sent in an alcohol solution when gout is being considered in the differential diagnosis. Similar to other types of inflammatory arthritis, synovial fluid white blood cell count (WBC) is typically elevated, frequently greater than 50,000 cells per mm^3 during an acute flare, making differentiation from a septic joint difficult.[13,14] Case series have reported concomitant septic and gouty arthritis exist with markedly elevated synovial WBC greater than 70,000/mm^3.[14,15] Serum uric acid levels add little information during an acute gout flare. Studies have found normal serum uric acid levels in 11% to 49% of patients during an acute flare, and these levels may actually decrease during the flare.[16,17] Thus, levels should be obtained during intercritical periods after resolution of the flare.

IMAGING EVALUATION

Radiographs play an important role in the evaluation of gout in the hand. Periarticular erosions with punched out or "rat-bite" lesions are common findings. Joint space narrowing is found in late disease (Fig. 2). Although the monosodium urate crystals are radiolucent themselves, the soft-tissue shadows that arise from tophi may be visible if of sufficient size (Fig. 3). An MRI may be helpful for evaluation of tophi of the flexor tendon sheath. MRI has been used to classify gout in the hand into a discrete nodular form, compartmental form, and a permeative form enveloping all structures across compartmental planes. Similarly, MRI has shown radiographs and physical examination underestimate the size and extent of tophi.[18] Dual-energy computed tomography (DECT) is a newer method to identify urate deposition by detecting material-specific differences in attenuation between calcium and urate when exposed to 2 different radiographic spectrums.[19] A diagnosis of gout by DECT is possible without crystal analysis in synovial fluid or tophi and without serum urate levels. Frequently, gouty deposition on DECT is portrayed on color-coded cross-sectional and 3-dimensional reconstructions for easy interpretation.

MEDICAL MANAGEMENT

Hyperuricemia reduction through lifestyle alteration as well as medical management serves to lessen or eliminate the incidence of painful acute gouty attacks and help lessen the severity of conditions that arise secondary to prolonged hyperuricemia. A trial period of nonoperative medical therapy should ideally precede surgical management of upper extremity gout manifestations.

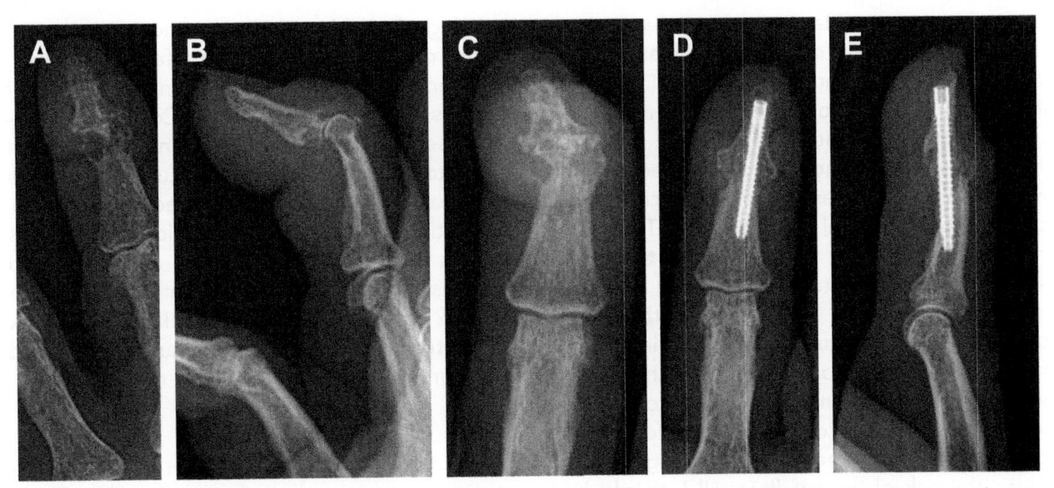

Fig. 2. (*A–C*) Patient with severe gouty arthritis of the distal interphalangeal joint (DIPJ). Plain films reveal periarticular erosions and flexion deformity of the DIPJ. (*D, E*) Arthrodesis of the DIPJ performed along with tophi excision. (*Courtesy of* Dr William J. Weller.)

Acute Gout Flare

An acute gout attack frequently presents as a sudden onset of extreme pain and swelling in an isolated region without antecedent trauma. Erythema, warmth, and motion limitation secondary to pain typically accompany acute flares and closely mimic infection. Pain frequently begins overnight during periods of lower body temperature. Patients report intense hypersensitivity to light touch or pressure over the affected part such as contact with a bed sheet. Joint immobilization and lifestyle modifications can reduce the discomfort but medical management is usually pivotal. The 2020 American College of Rheumatology (ACR) guidelines on the management of an acute gout flare recommend using colchicine, nonsteroidal antiinflammatory drugs (NSAIDs), or glucocorticoids (oral, intraarticular, or intramuscular) as first-line treatment.[20] The ACR does not recommend one over the other and states selection should be a shared decision with the patient based on past experience with a medication, medical comorbidities, and access to the medication. Frequent contraindications for NSAID use include renal disease, peptic ulcer disease, congestive heart failure, and anticoagulation therapy.[21] Colchicine administered for an acute gout flare starts at 1.2 mg followed by 0.6 mg an hour later.[20] It is then continued daily at 0.6 mg once or twice daily until flare resolution. Colchicine therapy may need be discontinued early due to gastrointestinal side effects, especially diarrhea, which are common with colchicine. Systemic corticosteroids should be considered with polyarticular involvement or in the setting of contraindications to NSAIDs.

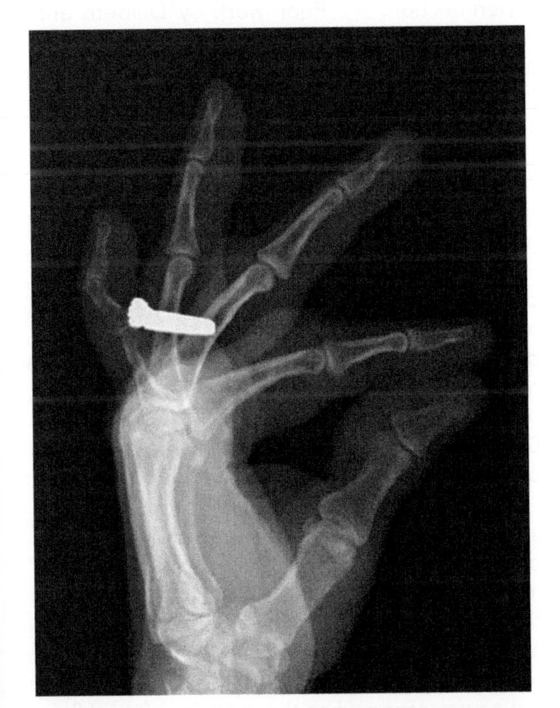

Fig. 3. Lateral radiograph of the left hand of patient in Fig. 5. Note the soft-tissue shadows visible over the proximal interphalangeal joints of index and middle fingers.

Chronic Pharmacologic Management

The ACR recommends pharmacologic urate lowering therapy (ULT) for patients with one or more subcutaneous tophi, radiographic damage due to gout, or 2 or more gout flares per year. They do not recommend ULT for asymptomatic hyperuricemia.[20] ULT should be initiated several weeks after an acute flare to prevent flare exacerbation. The 2 main classes of ULT are uricostatic and uricosuric agents. Uricostatic agents (allopurinol and febuxostat) block uric acid production through inhibition of xanthine oxidase, whereas uricosuric agents (probenecid and benzbromarone) increase urinary uric acid excretion by blocking renal reabsorption. The ACR strongly recommends allopurinol as the first-line agent for ULT, starting at a low dose of less than or equal to 100 mg/day with subsequent titration. Uricosuric agents are indicated for patients allergic to allopurinol with normal renal function. Antiinflammatory prophylaxis therapy with NSAIDs, colchicine, or systemic corticosteroids is indicated when initiating ULT to reduce the risk of a gout flare. ULT should be titrated to a target goal of serum uric acid level of less than 6 mg/dL.[20]

Lifestyle Modifications

Beyond pharmacologic treatment, dietary modifications are an important aspect in the management of gout. Alcohol intake has been shown to have a dose-dependent response with the incidence of gout with beer consumption having the greater impact over liquor. Moderate wine consumption did not increase the risk of gout.[22] Using data from almost 15,000 participants to assess the effect of purine-rich foods, serum uric acid levels increased with meat and seafood consumption. In contrast, dairy consumption was associated with a decrease in serum uric acid levels.[23] Purine rich vegetables were not associated with an increased risk of gout.[24] Choi and colleagues also demonstrated that higher body mass index and weight gain were risk factors for gout, whereas weight loss was a protective factor.[25] Patients with gout should be counseled to limit alcohol consumption, reduce purine-rich meats and seafood intake, and attempt weight loss.

CLINICAL MANIFESTATIONS AND SURGICAL TREATMENT

Gout has been called "the imitator" because it manifests itself in many ways in the hand and wrist that can be confused for other more common pathologies. Surgical treatment of gout in the hand is indicated only in a minority of patients. Straub and colleagues described the common categories of surgical indications for gout that are still used today: functional, symptomatic, and cosmetic.[26] Functional treatment includes excision or debulking of tophaceous gout to restore range of motion or permit the wearing of clothing. Symptomatic treatment includes controlling drainage or infection of tophi, decompression of nerves, or management of gout-associated arthropathy. Cosmetic treatment serves to restore a more normal appearance to unsightly tophi particularly in cases with dorsal hand tophi. Some recommend prophylactic administration of colchicine or NSAIDs 3 days before surgery for gout and continued administration 1 week postoperatively to reduce the risk of a postoperative gout flare.[27] The risk is greatest in patients with a presurgical uric acid level greater than or equal to 9 mg/dL.[28]

Tophi

Gouty tophi are typically the result of long-standing, uncontrolled hyperuricemia. Tophi may be found around the finger, wrist, and elbow joints. Tophi are most visible and palpable on the dorsum of the finger distal interphalangeal (DIP) joint but may also involve the proximal interphalangeal joint, metacarpophalangeal joint, extensor tendons on the dorsum of the hand, or rarely flexor tendons, or they may originate from the extensor tendons on the dorsum of the hand (Figs. 4 and 5). Skin overlying tophi may seem normal or exhibit a whitish hue in areas of thinner skin. With long-standing disease, tophi may ulcerate through the thin skin, leading to fistulas and superinfection.[26,29] Prior work by Dalbeth and colleagues demonstrated that tophi-associated arthropathy was an independent predictor of hand function.[30] Hand function diminishes as the size and number of tophi increase (see Fig. 5C). Patients with more than or equal to 1 tophus have also been shown to have decreased health-related quality-of-life scores and greater impairment of work productivity.[31]

As tophi of the hand may be both cosmetically displeasing and functionally limiting, treatment is often sought. ULT has been shown to diminish the size of tophi. A linear relationship has been established between the rate of tophi reduction and the mean serum urate level.[32] Dissolution of tophi may occur with correction of hyperuricemia through ULT.

Surgical management of symptomatic tophi includes tophus aspiration, open sharp excision or curettage, and intralesional shaving. Treatment is frequently dictated by the location of the tophi, whether closed or open techniques are desired, and if it is draining. Aspiration of a tophus at the DIP joint can be considered in the acute setting when the tophi is soft and fluctuant. Aspiration is performed with an 18-gauge needle through healthy appearing skin followed by manual expression of the gouty material.[33]

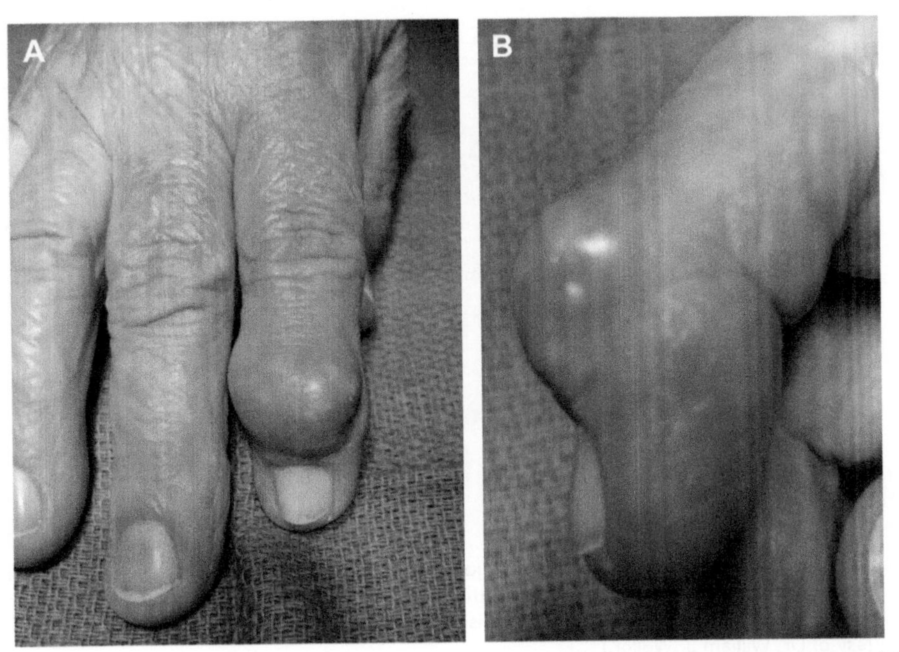

Fig. 4. Prominent tophus of the distal interphalangeal joint appreciated from the dorsal (*A*) and lateral (*B*) views.

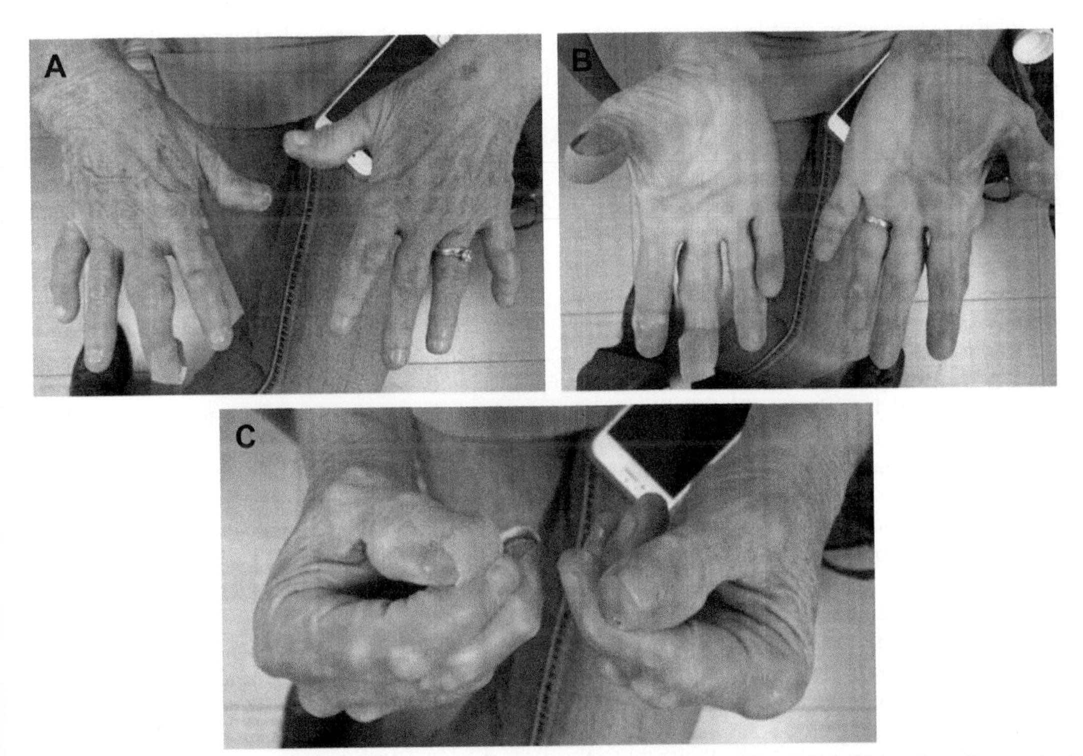

Fig. 5. Female patient with tophaceous gout of the bilateral hands. (*A*) Dorsal tophi are most visible at the proximal interphalangeal joint and metacarpophalangeal joints of the bilateral index and middle fingers. (*B*) Multiple volar finger pad tophi. Patient wore Band-Aids to cover drainage from the tophi. (*C*) Diminished finger flexion is appreciated with attempted grip.

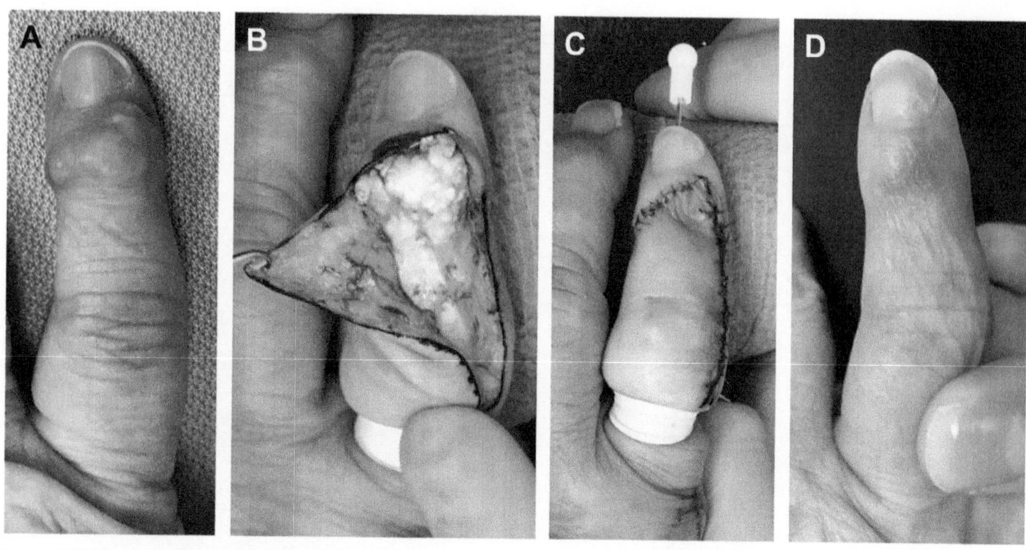

Fig. 6. (*A*) Gouty tophus of the distal interphalangeal joint (DIPJ) with white tophi visible. (*B*) A local advancement flap is elevated and tophi are exposed. (*C*) Burrow's triangle local advancement flap has been advanced distally, and the DIPJ has been temporarily pinned to detension the flap. (*D*) Good final cosmetic appearance of the DIPJ. (*Courtesy of* Dr. William J. Weller.)

Patients should continue with daily soaks in saline combined with manual tophus expression until no more can be expressed. The DIP joint should be splinted in extension for 4 weeks to control the extensor lag that is frequently seen.

Surgical resection, or tophectomy, typically involves an open approach to the tophus, raising healthy skin flaps, and directly shelling the urate lesion from the soft-tissue envelope and the underlying bone or tendons. Incisions should be carefully planned to avoid bony or tophi prominences where the thinned dermal microcirculation plexus may be impaired.[34] Curettes can be used to carefully dissect the tophus off native structures. Particular attention should be paid to handling of the soft tissues, as the skin covering is frequently tenuous.[20] Incisions should be closed loosely to allow fluid egress and avoid excessive flap pressure. At times, a local rotation advancement flap may be used to obtain more durable coverage (Fig. 6).

A soft-tissue shaver also has been used for debulking gouty tophi of the hand.[27,35,36] With this technique, a small shaver is introduced through multiple small portals in combination with a suction-irrigation system to debulk the gouty deposit. One of the primary goals of this technique is to minimize insult to the already tenuous soft-tissue envelope as would be expected with an open technique. Lee and colleagues reported their experience in 32 patients with tophi of the upper extremity.[35] They reported no major complications beyond 2 patients having an acute gout attack in the immediate postoperative period.

Chronic untreated tophi may eventually lead to skin ulceration and infection, prompting patients to seek medical attention. Rare cases of necrotizing fasciitis due to tophi have even been reported.[37] In a series of 131 patients with tophi, with 47% occurring in the hand, older age, larger tophus size, and lack of protective sensation were independent risk factors for ulceration.[38] Patients who develop infection at ulcerated tophi are older, have larger ulcer size, and longer ulcer duration.[39] A draining tophi sinus may present as intermittent pin-point drainage or continuous drainage. Ulceration may lead to bone or joint damage from osteomyelitis or septic arthritis. Ulceration may occur only at a small portion of the tophus. Curettage can be performed to debulk the tophi and relax the soft tissues to allow for better coverage to be obtained. Incisions should be extended from the margin of the ulcer, and counter-incisions should be made with caution due to the tenuous blood supply of the intervening skin. Skin grafting may be required in certain circumstances.[40]

Finger pad tophi are uncommon presentations for gouty tophi.[41] Finger pad tophi present as multiple small nodules or as a singular nodule on the volar distal phalanx of unknown cause. A broad differential diagnosis raises a diagnostic dilemma including benign tumors, malignant tumors, and mass lesions.[42] A thorough history to identify a preexisting diagnosis of gout and fine-needle aspiration cytology can aid in diagnosis. ULT can be initiated for smaller tophi, whereas surgical resection may be indicated for more rapid treatment of symptomatic finger pad tophi. Full-thickness skin graft may be required for reconstruction after resection of a superficial infiltrating tophus of the finger pad.[42]

Gouty Arthropathy

Gout is the number one world-wide cause of inflammatory arthropathy. Monosodium urate crystals, present within synovial fluid, undergo phagocytosis by macrophages leading to the downstream release of inflammatory mediators.[43] The long-standing inflammatory reaction progresses to cartilage erosion and articular damage as the gouty deposits invade the cartilage and subchondral bone[44]; this is most often seen affecting the DIP joint and is commonly found in combination with gouty tophi. Management involves conservative treatment with antiinflammatories and ULT. Surgical excision of the tophi may be all that is required to debulk the mass lesion. When conservative treatment fails, arthrodesis of the involved joint may be indicated (see Fig. 2).

Flexor Tenosynovitis and Trigger Finger

Flexor tenosynovitis is an atypical presentation of gout in the hands and can be easily misdiagnosed without a high index of suspicion.[45,46] Gouty flexor tenosynovitis can present as mobile nodules along the flexor tendons. Alternatively, diffuse infiltration of the flexor tendon by tophi may be present. Painful or painless reduction in digital range of motion can be seen. Localized involvement at the level of the A1 pulley can present as an atypical cause of trigger finger. Attritional tendon rupture may be present in rare cases. A thorough review of a patient's medical history for gout and laboratory evaluation of serum uric acid level will aid in diagnosis. Surgical exploration will reveal gouty tophi involving the flexor sheath and tendons. Tenosynovectomy of the involved tendons with debridement of tophi is the goal of surgical treatment. During the routine release of the A1 pulley for trigger finger, one may incidentally find gouty infiltration of the tendons.[47] Thorough tenosynovectomy is indicated to allow as much smooth tendon gliding as possible.

Finger Stiffness and Contractures

Digital flexion contractures can present as the end-stage result of gouty flexor tenosynovitis or large tophi (Fig. 7). Multiple cases have been reported on tophaceous deposits found within flexor tendons of the wrist, palm, and hand, leading to digital flexion contractures.[48–50] Patients may present with a fixed flexion deformity and report a history of triggering initially. A mass may or may not be palpable. Flexor tendon tophaceous infiltration

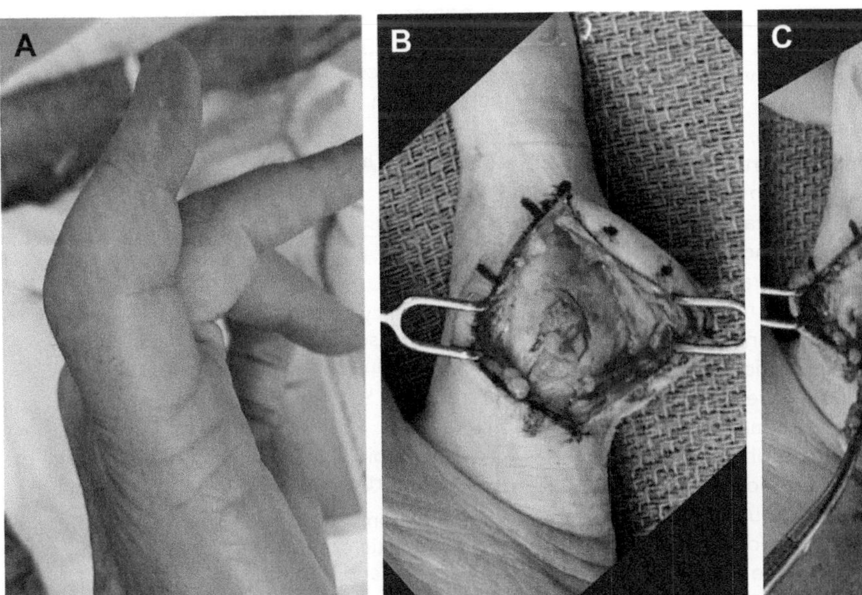
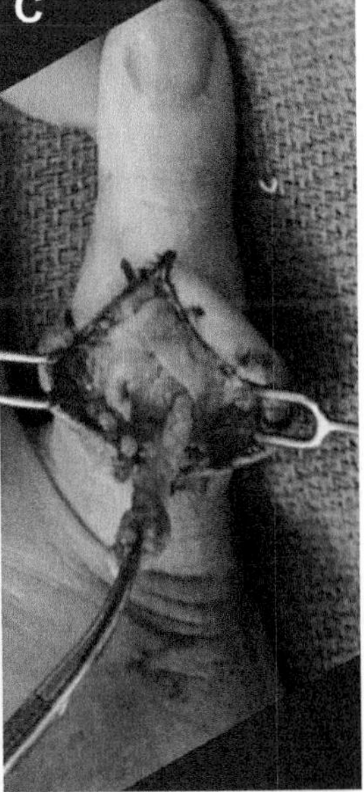

Fig. 7. (A) Flexion contracture of the proximal interphalangeal joint (B) Gouty tophi have erupted through the central slip (C) Excision of the tophus material from the dorsal proximal interphalangeal joint.

proximal to the carpal tunnel may present with isolated digital flexion due to the inability of the tendon to glide through the flexor retinaculum.[51,52] Advanced imaging with MRI identifies structures involved and their locations. Surgery involves debridement of the white tophi deposits from the flexor tendons to attempt to improve tendon gliding. Tendons can be encased with gout, and resection of a portion of the tendon may be required. Sacrifice of one or both of the flexor tendons may be required, and tendon grafting may be indicated for later reconstruction. Medical management with ULT is also recommended to reduce serum urate levels and the risk of recurrence especially if delayed flexor tendon reconstruction efforts are to be attempted.

Neural Compression

Tophaceous gout can increase the volume of the carpal tunnel, leading to median nerve compression and ultimately carpal tunnel syndrome. Multiple case reports have described gouty deposits found within the flexor tendons crossing the carpal tunnel or along the walls of the canal.[50,53–55] Treatment involves release of the transverse carpal ligament and other compressive structures, debridement of tophi, and tenosynovectomy to decrease the contents within the carpal tunnel. Resection of highly infiltrated tendons may be required. Hence, urate crystal deposition should be included in the differential diagnosis for carpal tunnel syndrome, especially in men with a history of gout.[54]

Gout of the Wrist

Beyond affecting the traversing flexor and extensor tendons at the wrist, gout can also occur within the carpus, albeit rare. Carpal involvement may lead to formation of cartilage erosions, lytic lesions, and periarticular damage that are visible on radiographs.[56,57] Most cases can be treated medically with urate-lowering therapy. In severe cases, curettage and bone grafting of lytic lesions or wrist arthrodesis may be necessary.[20] Intraarticular soft-tissue involvement also has been reported, with crystal deposition identified on the scapholunate and lunotriquetral ligaments.[58–60] In this setting the articular cartilage wear follows the pattern seen in scapholunate advanced collapse.[58] There is little evidence for treatment of ligament disruption in gout, but, again, medical treatment is recommended. Although ligament reconstruction can be considered in the setting of scapholunate dissociation with preserved articular surfaces, bony procedures are probably more predictable.

SUMMARY

Gout frequently affects the hands of patients usually after periods of long-standing hyperuricemia. The mainstay of treatment involves urate lowering therapy to decrease the risk of gout flares and the size of symptomatic tophi. Surgical indications as discussed earlier are to increase functional capability through pain reduction, improvement in motion, and improvement in cosmetic appearance.

Gout frequently imitates other more common pathologies of the hand, and the surgeon should remain vigilant to this diagnosis in patients with a history of gout. Common hand conditions, such as trigger finger and carpal tunnel syndrome in patients relatively asymptomatic from their premorbid gout condition, may have somewhat unusual findings at surgery. Hence, routinely reviewing the patient's medical history before surgical intervention may lessen the likelihood of a surprise intraoperative surgical finding in a patient with gout.

Although gout is certainly more frequently associated with the great toe, upper extremity involvement may be the sole reason a patient seeks orthopedic evaluation. Not infrequently, an upper extremity surgeon may be the first health care provider to see a patient with undiagnosed gout. When indicated, a prescription of oral steroids, NSAIDs such as a short course of indomethacin, colchicine, or an intraarticular steroid injection may provide prompt and satisfactory pain relief. Working in conjunction with a primary care provider such as an internist or rheumatologist is recommended to maximize medical recovery, if possible, before surgical intervention.

CLINICS CARE POINTS

- Lifestyle alteration lessens the severity and frequency of gout attacks. Patients should be counseled to limit alcohol consumption and purine-rich meats and seafood and attempt weight loss.
- For an acute gout flare-up, colchicine, nonsteroidal antiinflammatory medication, or glucocorticoids are first-line treatments.
- For chronic gout, urate-lowering therapy with uricostatic or uricosuric agents is recommended.
- Symptomatic treatment and urate-lowering therapy are frequently all that is required for management of most upper extremity gout.

- Surgical management of symptomatic tophi includes aspiration, open sharp excision or curettage, and intralesional shaving, depending on location, ulceration, drainage, or infection.
- Arthrodesis of the involved joint may be necessary in gouty arthropathy.
- For the atypical presentation of flexor tenosynovitis, tenosynovectomy with debridement of tophi is the goal of surgical treatment.
- If tophaceous gout increases the volume of the carpal tunnel, leading to median nerve compression, release of the transverse ligament and other compressive structures, tophi debridement, and tenosynovectomy may be necessary.

DISCLOSURE

The authors have no disclosures and report no conflicts of interest in regard to this manuscript.

REFERENCES

1. Mikuls TR, Farrar JT, Bilker WB, et al. Gout epidemiology: results from the UK General Practice Research Database, 1990-1999. Ann Rheum Dis 2005;64(2):267–72.
2. Roddy E, Choi HK. Epidemiology of gout. Rheum Dis Clin North Am 2014;40(2):155–75.
3. Singh G, Lingala B, Mithal A. Gout and hyperuricaemia in the USA: prevalence and trends. Rheumatology (Oxford) 2019;58(12):2177–80.
4. Eun Y, Kim IY, Han K, et al. Association between female reproductive factors and gout: a nationwide population-based cohort study of 1 million postmenopausal women. Arthritis Res Ther 2021;23(1):304.
5. Mallinson PI, Reagan AC, Coupal T, et al. The distribution of urate deposition within the extremities in gout: a review of 148 dual-energy CT cases. Skeletal Radiol 2014;43(3):277–81.
6. Dalbeth N, Merriman TR, Stamp LK. Gout Lancet 2016;388(10055):2039–52.
7. Perez-Ruiz F, Calabozo M, Erauskin GG, et al. Renal underexcretion of uric acid is present in patients with apparent high urinary uric acid output. Arthritis Rheum 2002;47(6):610–3.
8. Meller M, Epstein A, Meller AY, et al. Hyperuricemia and gout in orthopaedics. J Bone Joint Surg Rev 2018;6(10):e11.
9. Campion EW, Glynn RJ, DeLabry LO. Asymptomatic hyperuricemia. Risks and consequences in the Normative Aging Study. Am J Med 1987;82(3):421–6.
10. Bhole V, de Vera M, Rahman MM, et al. Epidemiology of gout in women: Fifty-two-year followup of a prospective cohort. Arthritis Rheum 2010;62(4):1069–76.
11. Shoji A, Yamanaka H, Kamatani N. A retrospective study of the relationship between serum urate level and recurrent attacks of gouty arthritis: evidence for reduction of recurrent gouty arthritis with antihyperuricemic therapy. Arthritis Rheum 2004;51(3):321–5.
12. Pascual E, Batlle-Gualda E, Martínez A, et al. Synovial fluid analysis for diagnosis of intercritical gout. Ann Intern Med 1999;131(10):756–9.
13. Krey PR, Bailen DA. Synovial fluid leukocytosis. A study of extremes. Am J Med 1979;67(3):436–42.
14. Luo TD, Jarvis DL, Yancey HB, et al. Synovial cell count poorly predicts septic arthritis in the presence of crystalline arthropathy. J Bone Jt Infect 2020;5(3):118–24.
15. Shah K, Spear J, Nathanson LA, et al. Does the presence of crystal arthritis rule out septic arthritis? J Emerg Med 2007;32(1):23–6.
16. Leiszler M, Poddar S, Fletcher A. Clinical inquiry. Are serum uric acid levels always elevated in acute gout? J Fam Pract 2011;60(10):618–20.
17. Logan JA, Morrison E, McGill PE. Serum uric acid in acute gout. Ann Rheum Dis 1997;56(11):696–7.
18. Popp JD, Bidgood WD Jr, Edwards NL. Magnetic resonance imaging of tophaceous gout in the hands and wrists. Semin Arthritis Rheum 1996;25(4):282–9.
19. Desai MA, Peterson JJ, Garner HW, et al. Clinical utility of dual-energy CT for evaluation of tophaceous gout. Radiographics 2011;31(5):1365–77.
20. FitzGerald JD, Dalbeth N, Mikuls T, et al. American College of Rheumatology Guideline for the Management of Gout [published correction appears in. Arthritis Care Res (Hoboken) 2020;72(8):1187 [published correction appears in Arthritis Care Res (Hoboken). 2021 Mar;73(3):458]. Arthritis Care Res (Hoboken). 2020;72(6):744-760. doi:10.1002/acr.24180.
21. Fitzgerald BT, Setty A, Mudgal CS. Gout affecting the hand and wrist. J Am Acad Orthop Surg 2007;15(10):625–35.
22. Choi HK, Atkinson K, Karlson EW, et al. Alcohol intake and risk of incident gout in men: a prospective study. Lancet 2004;363(9417):1277–81.
23. Choi HK, Liu S, Curhan G. Intake of purine-rich foods, protein, and dairy products and relationship to serum levels of uric acid: the Third National Health and Nutrition Examination Survey. Arthritis Rheum 2005;52(1):283–9.
24. Choi HK, Atkinson K, Karlson EW, et al. Purine-rich foods, dairy and protein intake, and the risk of gout in men. N Engl J Med 2004;350(11):1093–103.
25. Choi HK, Atkinson K, Karlson EW, et al. Obesity, weight change, hypertension, diuretic use, and risk of gout in men: the health professionals follow-up study. Arch Intern Med 2005;165(7):742–8.

26. Straub LR, Smith JW, Carpenter GK, et al. The surgery of gout in the upper extremity. J Bone Joint Surg 1961;43(5):731–74.
27. Lee SS, Lin SD, Lai CS, et al. The soft-tissue shaving procedure for deformity management of chronic tophaceous gout. Ann Plast Surg 2003;51(4):372–5.
28. Jeong H, Jeon CH. Clinical characteristics and risk factors for gout flare during the postsurgical period. Adv Rheumatol 2019;59(1):31.
29. Bouaziz W, Rekik MA, Guidara AR, et al. Infection of a tophaceous nodule of the wrist and hand. BMJ Case Rep 2018;2018. bcr2018226029.
30. Dalbeth N, Collis J, Gregory K, et al. Tophaceous joint disease strongly predicts hand function in patients with gout. Rheumatology (Oxford) 2007;46(12):1804–7.
31. Khanna PP, Nuki G, Bardin T, et al. Tophi and frequent gout flares are associated with impairments to quality of life, productivity, and increased healthcare resource use: Results from a cross-sectional survey. Health Qual Life Outcomes 2012;10:117.
32. Perez-Ruiz F, Calabozo M, Pijoan JI, et al. Effect of urate-lowering therapy on the velocity of size reduction of tophi in chronic gout. Arthritis Rheum 2002;47(4):356–60.
33. Mudgal CS. Management of tophaceous gout of the distal interphalangeal joint. J Hand Surg Br 2006;31(1):101–3.
34. Doscher M, Beutel BG, Lovy A, et al. En masse excision and curettage for periarticular gouty tophi of the hands. Eplasty 2022;22:e25.
35. Lee SS, Sun IF, Lu YM, et al. Surgical treatment of the chronic tophaceous deformity in upper extremities - the shaving technique. J Plast Reconstr Aesthet Surg 2009;62(5):669–74.
36. Lee SS, Chen MC, Chou YH, et al. Timing of intralesion shaving for surgical treatment of chronic tophus. J Plast Reconstr Aesthet Surg 2013;66(8):1131–7.
37. Yu KH, Ho HH, Chen JY, et al. Gout complicated with necrotizing fasciitis–report of 15 cases. Rheumatology (Oxford) 2004;43(4):518–21.
38. Xu J, Lin C, Zhang P, et al. Risk factors for ulceration over tophi in patients with gout. Int Wound J 2017; 14(4):704–7.
39. Xu J, Zhu Z, Zhang W. Clinical characteristics of infectious ulceration over tophi in patients with gout. J Int Med Res 2018;46(6):2258–64.
40. Larmon WA. Surgical management of tophaceous gout. Clin Orthop Relat Res 1970;71:56–69.
41. Holland NW, Jost D, Beutler A, et al. Finger pad tophi in gout. J Rheumatol 1996;23(4):690–2.
42. Bera S, Sharma S, Gupta V, et al. Management of ulcerated finger pad tophi. Reumatologia 2020; 58(3):173–8.
43. Martinon F, Pétrilli V, Mayor A, et al. Gout-associated uric acid crystals activate the NALP3 inflammasome. Nature 2006;440(7081):237–41.
44. Meyer Zu Reckendorf G, Dahmam A. Hand involvement in gout [published online ahead of print, 2018 May 17]. Hand Surg Rehabil 2018;S2468-1229(18): 30065–73.
45. Moore JR, Weiland AJ. Gouty tenosynovitis in the hand. J Hand Surg Am 1985;10(2):291–5.
46. Weniger FG, Davison SP, Risin M, et al. Gouty flexor tenosynovitis of the digits: report of three cases. J Hand Surg Am 2003;28(4):669–72.
47. Doucet V, McLeod GJ, Petropolis CJ. Gouty stenosing tenosynovitis: trigger finger as a first presentation of tophaceous gout. Plast Reconstr Surg Glob Open 2020;8(8):e3055.
48. Caudle RJ, Heim JM, Stern PJ. Digital flexion contractures secondary to tophaceous gout. A report of three cases. Orthopedics 1989;12(5):731–5.
49. Kumar R, Sahni VK, Jauhar S. Finger flexion contracture: first manifestation of gout. J Orthop Case Rep 2015;5(2):66–8.
50. Hernández-Cortés P, Caba M, Gómez-Sánchez R, et al. Digital flexion contracture and severe carpal tunnel syndrome due to tophaceus infiltration of wrist flexor tendon: first manifestation of gout. Orthopedics 2011;34(11):e797–9.
51. Chieng D, Ang X, Teoh C, et al. Atypical trigger finger: first manifestation of gout. Open J Orthopedics 2018;8:423–8.
52. Sano K, Kohakura Y, Kimura K, et al. Atypical triggering at the wrist due to intratendinous infiltration of tophaceous gout. Hand (N Y). 2009;4(1): 78–80.
53. Mockford BJ, Kincaid RJ, Mackay I. Carpal tunnel syndrome secondary to intratendinous infiltration by tophaceous gout. Scand J Plast Reconstr Surg Hand Surg 2003;37(3):186–7.
54. Rich JT, Bush DC, Lincoski CJ, et al. Carpal tunnel syndrome due to tophaceous gout. Orthopedics 2004;27(8):862–3.
55. Carr L, Brooke S, Ingraham J. Medically managed gout precipitating acute carpal tunnel syndrome. Hand (N Y). 2015;10(3):574–7.
56. Jerome JT, Sankaran B, Thirumagal K. Carpal bone involvement in gout. Arch Orthop Trauma Surg 2007;127(10):971–4.
57. Poelzer C, Hildebrand KA. Gout of the wrist. J Am Soc Surg Hand 2004;4(4):256–65.
58. Wilcznski MC, Gelberman RH, Adams A, et al. Arthroscopic findings in gout of the wrist. J Hand Surg 2009;34(2):244–50.
59. Ohishi T, Koide Y, Takahashi M, et al. Scapholunate dissociation caused by gouty arthritis of the wrist. Case Report Scand J Plast Reconstr Surg Hand Surg 2000;34(2):189–91.
60. Helfgott SM, Skoff H. Scapholunate dissociation associated with crystal induced synovitis. J Rheumatol 1992;19(3):485–7.

Shoulder and Elbow

Understanding Medical Optimization for Patients Undergoing Shoulder Arthroplasty

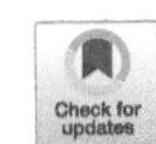

Jessica L. Churchill, MD, Conner J. Paez, MD,
Vahid Entezari, MD, Eric T. Ricchetti, MD,
Jason C. Ho, MD*

KEYWORDS

- Preoperative optimization • Medical optimization • Total shoulder arthroplasty
- Reverse total shoulder arthroplasty • Preoperative care • Surgical planning

KEY POINTS

- Medical optimization of comorbidities before total shoulder arthroplasty is important in order to improve outcomes, reduce complications, and reduce costs.
- Appropriate preoperative screening should include a comprehensive assessment of the patient including physical examination, laboratory evaluation, medication review, and social/behavioral evaluation.
- Diabetes, anemia, preoperative medication, malnutrition, and social/behavioral considerations such as depression, opioid use, and smoking can be managed and optimized before surgery.

BACKGROUND

Total shoulder arthroplasty (TSA) is an effective and common treatment of end-stage glenohumeral joint pathologic condition and is associated with excellent long-term outcomes. In the last 2 decades, there have been dramatic increases in surgical volume for TSA,[1] and predictive models show an expected increase of more than 200% by 2025.[2] Additionally, a wider variety of patients, including older patients, is now undergoing TSA. As the rate of TSA increases, especially in older patient groups, so does the overall number of complications. Although outcomes of TSA are generally excellent, complication rates have ranged from 2.8% to 12% in recent studies.[1,3,4] When complications do occur after TSA, they can be devastating for the patient and incur great costs to the health-care system.

In an effort to reduce the risk of complications after TSA, many surgeons seek to optimize their patients' comorbid conditions preoperatively. Literature has shown that assessing, risk stratifying, and medically optimizing patients before surgery can help lower postoperative complication rates.[5,6] To effectively optimize patients before TSA, the surgeon should be familiar with recognizing and treating common medical comorbidities found in orthopedic patients including anemia, diabetes, malnutrition, cardiovascular conditions, and history of deep venous thrombosis.[7] Although preoperative optimization is often aimed at older patients, even younger, healthy patients can be optimized to reduce potential complications. Current literature is mostly based in total hip and knee arthroplasty or other surgical subspecialties; however, in this review, we attempt to examine this topic

Cleveland Clinic Foundation, Department of Orthopaedic Surgery, A40, 9500 Euclid Avenue, Cleveland, OH 44195, USA
* Corresponding author.
E-mail address: Hoj@ccf.org

Orthop Clin N Am 54 (2023) 309–318
https://doi.org/10.1016/j.ocl.2023.02.004
0030-5898/23/

with the existing TSA literature to make preoperative optimization recommendations for TSA.

PATIENT EVALUATION OVERVIEW

Preoperative evaluation and medical optimization are critical to improving patient outcomes after TSA surgery. This consists of identifying and treating modifiable patient and environmental risk factors that may affect postoperative outcomes.[7] Dlott and colleagues compared 463 patients undergoing total knee arthroplasty that were enrolled or not enrolled in a presurgical optimization program, finding that medical optimization of patients before total joint surgery decreases average length of stay (LOS), return emergency department (ED) visits, and percentage of patients discharged to a location other than home.[7,8] This underscores the importance of addressing modifiable risk factors before taking a patient to the operating room for an elective joint replacement procedure such as TSA.

A thorough history and physical examination should be the cornerstone of any preoperative optimization plan. This assessment should guide the decision to order laboratory testing. Although not every patient needs an extensive laboratory workup, studies have agreed there are a few essential laboratory tests every presurgical patient should receive.[9] These include a complete blood count (CBC) and a basic metabolic panel. Patient comorbidities should guide additional testing such as a hemoglobin A1c for prediabetic or diabetic patients. Older patients or those with active cardiac signs or symptoms should have an electrocardiogram (EKG) performed. Literature has shown that patients should also have EKG testing if they are undergoing an intermediate risk procedure, such as TSA, with at least one of the following risk factors: ischemic heart disease, congestive heart failure (CHF), cerebrovascular disease, insulin-dependent diabetes, or a preoperative creatinine greater than 2.0 mg/mL.[7] Further cardiac workup by an internal medicine physician, anesthesiologist, or cardiologist may be necessary based on the results of initial cardiac screening.

Medication lists should also be carefully scrutinized before surgery because many medications may have adverse effects perioperatively. Some medications, such as anticoagulants, disease-modifying antirheumatic drugs, and steroids, may need to be adjusted or withheld during the perioperative period. Close communication between surgeons and the other physicians and care team members is critical to balance risk versus reward when changing or holding medications or treatment plans during the perioperative period.

Similarly, a patient's social and behavioral health is tied to outcomes after surgery. Studies have shown that depression, anxiety, and other mental health issues can significantly affect a patient's recovery and postoperative course; therefore, it is prudent to consider these disorders when conducting the history and physical before surgery.[10–13] Similar to medical comorbidities, these issues can often be optimized before surgery. A very significant social risk factor for adverse events after TSA is smoking, and this social determinant of health can be effectively intervened on before surgery. Functional status should also be appropriately assessed before surgery, particularly ambulatory dysfunction because this can affect mobility, limit compliance with postoperative restrictions, and increase fall risk. In a study by Sridharan and colleagues, shoulder arthroplasty patients had a fall rate of 10.6% in the 90-day period postoperatively.[14] Patients with ambulatory difficulty preoperatively are more likely to require discharge to a location other than home and require a longer LOS after surgery. Taking a holistic approach to patient preoperative optimization helps ensure the maximum benefit is achieved in terms of postoperative outcomes.

After thorough assessment of the patient, initial laboratory result review, medication list scrutiny, and social/behavioral evaluation, decisions can be made regarding steps to medically optimize the patient before surgery.

PHARMACOLOGIC OR MEDICAL TREATMENT OPTIONS

After initial evaluation of a patient and identification of modifiable risk factors, a plan must be made to appropriately manage the patient's comorbidities in the perioperative period. Medical complications comprise 82% of 90-day readmissions after primary shoulder arthroplasty[15]; therefore, it is important to optimize the medical conditions of patients, when possible, before surgery. Medical optimization aims to limit complications and readmissions after shoulder arthroplasty.

COMMON COMORBIDITIES AND GOALS FOR OPTIMIZATION

Diabetes

Although diabetes is prevalent throughout the general population, it is even more common in surgical patients.[16] Patients with diabetes account for an estimated 10% to 20% of all surgical patients, and an estimated 23% to 60% of surgical patients have undiagnosed diabetes.[16,17] Mahure and colleagues examined 44,050 patients undergoing primary TSA and found diabetes was an independent risk factor for nonhome bound discharge, LOS in 75th percentile, total charges in the 75th percentile, and postoperative acute renal failure.[18] Scott and colleagues confirmed diabetes to be a significant risk factor for 90-day readmission after TSA.[19] Due to the increased complication risk in patients undergoing TSA with diabetes, it is important to include glycemic screening and management in the preoperative optimization of patients.

Measurement of the Hemoglobin A_{1c} (HbA_{1c}) level is generally accepted as the most appropriate screening test for hyperglycemia.[20] Although there are many accepted tests to diagnose diabetes, an HbA_{1c} test is easier and more convenient for patients than a fasting blood glucose or oral glucose tolerance test, and the result is less affected by day-to-day variability.[16,20] A preoperative HbA_{1c} level of greater than 7.0% requires preoperative optimization, and these patients should be referred to their primary care physician or an endocrinologist for optimization to a target blood glucose level of 5 to 10 mmol/L.[16] Controlling hyperglycemia preoperatively can mitigate the increased risk of postoperative complications faced by patients with diabetes.[16] Literature for lower extremity total joint arthroplasty recommends a preoperative HbA_{1c} of less than 7.5%.[21] In terms of TSA, Cancienne and colleagues demonstrated that patients with diabetes had significantly higher rates of wound complication and deep infection. They also found that there was an inflection point at HbA_{1c} greater than 8.0 where patients had dramatic increase in wound complications and postoperative deep infection requiring surgical intervention.[22] McElvaney and colleagues found that patients with diabetes undergoing elective TSA had significantly higher risk of 90-day readmission compared with those without diabetes but did not find an association between diabetes severity and other postoperative complications.[23] Overall, given the high rate of undiagnosed diabetes and prediabetes in surgical patients, patients undergoing TSA should be considered for diabetes screening with a HbA_{1c} if no recent HbA_{1c} is available so that treatment may be initiated because there are clear benefits of perioperative glycemic control.[16,22,23]

Cardiac

In TSA research, a history of cardiac disease has been shown to be one of the most important independent variables significantly associated with any complication.[24] Waterman and colleagues reported that cardiac disease was an independent predictor of mortality in their retrospective review of 2004 patients undergoing elective TSA.[25] Additionally, Farng and colleagues retrospectively reviewed 15,288 patients who underwent primary TSA and hemiarthroplasty during a 10-year period and found that cardiac disease was independently associated with a complication within 90 days of surgery.[26] Most physicians agree that a preoperative EKG is necessary in any patient aged older than 65 years before undergoing elective surgery such as TSA, especially for those with a history of cardiac disease.[27] Furthermore, it may be prudent to work closely with the patient's cardiologist in the preoperative period to ensure they are safe for surgery.

In addition to a preoperative EKG, preoperative B-type natriuretic peptide (BNP) levels can predict short-term and long-term postoperative cardiac events in orthopedic surgery patients.[28] BNP levels are commonly used to monitor patients with CHF, a known risk factor for postoperative complications in TSA.[29] Breidthardt and colleagues determined good predictive accuracy of preoperative BNP screening in orthopedic patients. They found the area under curve determining the potential of BNP to predict long-term cardiac events was 0.71. Additionally, with an optimal, calculated BNP threshold of 145 pg/mL, sensitivity and specificity were 53% and 90%.[28] Clinicians may consider ordering a preoperative BNP in patients undergoing TSA as part of a comprehensive preoperative optimization protocol.

Anemia

The World Health Organization defines anemia as a hemoglobin level less than 120 g/L in women and less than 130 g/L in men or a hematocrit less than 36% in women and 40% in men.[30] These definitions have been validated by large population studies examining mean hemoglobin values by age, race, and sex.[16,31] Orthopedic surgery populations have been shown to contain a strikingly high rate of anemia (25%–44%).[16,32] This is concerning because preoperative anemia is associated with increased infectious complication rates in total joint replacement patients.[16,33]

Doan and colleagues examined patients undergoing TSA specifically to determine the effects of preoperative anemia.[34] They found increasing severity of anemia to be associated with progressively worse 30-day postoperative outcomes. Of the 15,185 patients included in their study, 11,404 had normal hematocrit levels, 2962 patients were mildly anemic, and 819 patients had moderate-to-severe anemia. The found that with increasing severity of anemia, there was an increased average hospital LOS, rate of readmissions, and rate of all reoperations. In fact, multivariate analysis identified anemia as an independent predictor of readmissions, reoperations, minor complications, and major complications.[34] This points to preoperative anemia as an important intervention area to help optimize patient outcomes after TSA.

Hemoglobin levels, as determined by a CBC, represent the gold standard diagnostic test for anemia.[16] Additionally, obtaining a ferritin level should also be considered because iron-deficiency anemia is the most common cause of anemia in patients undergoing surgery.[16] A serum ferritin level less than 30 μg/L has been shown to be both sensitive (92%) and specific (98%) for the diagnosis of iron deficiency anemia.[35] Iron supplementation either orally or intravenously is the treatment of choice for iron deficiency anemia; however, many orthopedic surgeons may not wish to oversee treatment themselves and refer patients screening positive for preoperative anemia to their primary care physician for optimization.[16,35] Overall, there is sufficient evidence from high-quality trials to inform recommendations for the diagnosis and management of preoperative anemia; therefore, routine screening, investigation and treatment of preoperative anemia should be included in the preoperative optimization process for any patient being assessed for TSA.[16]

Anticoagulation

Anticoagulation medication is becoming increasingly prevalent in the surgical population. Managing both anticoagulation and antiplatelet medication preoperatively is important to limit the risk of significant postoperative complications. An elevated international normalized ration (INR) greater than 1.8 is a major risk factor for postoperative surgical site hemorrhage, whereas an INR ratio of 1.3 or 1.4 is considered safe and is associated with reduced postoperative and intraoperative bleeding.[7] Traditionally, the practice has been to discontinue warfarin and manage perioperative anticoagulation with 3 different methods: no treatment, low–molecular-weight heparin (LMWH), or heparin, depending on patient risk.[7] In low-risk patients undergoing elective orthopedic surgery, warfarin can be discontinued 5 days before surgery to achieve a target INR of less than 1.3. Patients at high or intermediate risk for developing a venous thromboembolism (VTE) or arterial thromboembolism during this period may be candidates for bridging therapy. LMWH and unfractionated heparin are the 2 main pharmacologic options for bridging therapy, and both should be stopped within 24 hours of planned surgery.[7]

Patients who are on antiplatelet therapy should also have a discussion with their surgeon about perioperative medication management before TSA. The use of the antiplatelet medication clopidogrel bisulfate has been increasing, especially in patients with drug-eluting or non-eluting cardiac stents.[36] Aspirin and clopidogrel are commonly used in combination in patients with acute coronary syndrome.[7] Due to an increase in the rate of stent thrombosis, elective surgery should be avoided in patients on clopidogrel bisulfate in the first 6 months after stent placement.[37] For patients on dual therapy, a perioperative management plan should be developed with their cardiologist. For patients on aspirin alone, literature from lower extremity arthroplasty has shown it is safe to operate without discontinuation of aspirin; however, each surgeon must assess their comfortability as lower extremity literature cannot be directly applied to upper extremity procedures.[38,39] Conversely, Rogers and colleagues examined patients undergoing TSA on clopidogrel and found significantly greater intraoperative blood loss and 90-day complication rates when clopidogrel was continued through surgery.[40] Surgeons should consider holding clopidogrel preoperatively in light of these findings. Previous literature has suggested preoperative hold intervals of 7 to 10 days.[36,37] In general, if the operating surgeon is uncertain about individual patients' risks of pausing anticoagulation, it is prudent to consult vascular medicine or cardiology for guidance perioperatively.

Malnutrition

Malnutrition, defined in literature as an albumin level less than 3.5 g/dL, is a common medical comorbidity that has been previously associated with poor postoperative outcomes across other surgical fields, including general surgery, vascular surgery, and transplant surgery.[41] In orthopedics, malnutrition has been associated with poor outcomes after total joint surgery, including major postoperative medical complications, delayed postoperative recovery, poor wound healing, increased hospital LOS, infection, and wound drainage.[41,42] Flamant and colleagues examined 421 primary and 71 revision elective shoulder arthroplasty cases looking at preoperative albumin and postoperative outcomes.[41] Interestingly, they found a 36.6% malnutrition rate in revision patients undergoing TSA and a 19.5% rate in primary patients undergoing TSA, making malnutrition a more prevalent problem than many surgeons would anticipate.[41] They found that patients undergoing primary shoulder arthroplasty with low-preoperative albumin levels defined as less than 3.5 g/dL have an increased risk of extended LOS after surgery.[41] Padegimas and colleagues found nutritional deficiency/weight loss to be associated with prosthetic joint infection (PJI) after shoulder arthroplasty with an odds ratio (OR) of 2.62.[43] This was the strongest positive predictor for PJI of all medical comorbidities analyzed in that study, which included others such as diabetes, drug abuse, anemia, heart failure, and pulmonary disease among others. Garcia and colleagues found that in patients undergoing TSA, malnutrition was significantly associated with increased risk for pulmonary complications, anemia requiring transfusion, and mortality.[44]

After the identification of preoperative malnutrition, the question remains whether correction in the form of nutritional supplementation improves postoperative outcomes. Currently, systematic reviews and meta-analyses representing several nonorthopedic surgical fields have found that nutritional repletion preoperatively reduces postoperative complications.[41,45,46] Based on this body of literature, it is reasonable to refer patients undergoing TSA with preoperative malnutrition to a dietitian for supplementation before surgery.

Obesity

Overweight, obesity, and morbid obesity are generally defined as a body mass index (BMI) of 25 kg/m^2 or greater, 30 kg/m^2 or greater, and 40 kg/m^2 or greater, respectively. Overweight and obesity have become a global health crisis during recent decades with wide reaching effects in all aspects of health care. It has been estimated that the rates of overweight and obesity have increased by 27.5% in adults and 47.1% in children between 1980 and 2013.[47] In 2013, 36.9% of men and 38.0% of women were considered overweight.[47] The increasing rates of overweight and obesity is a pattern that has been prevalent in both developed and developing countries, highlighting its global significance. The effects of obesity have been well studied in lower extremity arthroplasty with a large multitude of studies demonstrating the impact of obesity of postoperative outcomes, most notably superficial infection, deep infection, dislocation, and patient reported outcome scores.[48–50] There has been significantly less volume of literature on the impact of obesity on upper extremity arthroplasty. One study performed by Wagner and colleagues analyzed the effect of BMI as a continuous variable in shoulder arthroplasty implant survival and complication rates. It was found that increasing BMI was associated with increasing risk of revision surgical procedure, reoperation, revision for mechanical failure, and superficial infection.[51] Other studies have not found as strong of an effect, however. Anakwenze and colleagues found that increasing BMI was marginally associated with increased risk for 90-day readmission in TSA and marginally associated with higher risk of 3-year deep infection in reverse TSA.[51] Overall, it seems that obesity has at the very least some impact on patient outcomes after orthopedic procedures, including shoulder arthroplasty. Patients should be counseled preoperatively on their risk for complications if obese and appropriate management or referral should be considered to optimize these risks.

Vitamin D Deficiency

Most literature defines vitamin D deficiency as a serum 25-hydroxyvitamin D level less than 32 ng/mL.[52] Vitamin D deficiency has been associated with chronic health conditions and is present in about 40% of the general population, and there is a known high prevalence of vitamin D deficiency in patients undergoing orthopedic surgery.[52] Smith and colleagues examined 1674 vitamin D-deficient patients undergoing TSA and found a significantly higher rate of revision in the vitamin D-deficient patients compared with 5022 control patients.[52] There is a significant and well-documented risk for acromial stress fracture after reverse TSA in patients with osteopenia and osteoporosis, underlining the importance of bone health and adequate vitamin D levels in patients undergoing TSA.[53,54] Additional literature has shown that active treatment with vitamin D supplementation and maintenance of normal serum levels should be considered for better postoperative functional outcome and quality of life after orthopedic surgery.[55,56] Measuring a patient's serum 25-hydroxyvitamin D preoperatively and treating deficiencies, if necessary, could be considered in a preoperative optimization protocol before TSA.

NONPHARMACOLOGIC OR SURGICAL/ INTERVENTIONAL TREATMENT OPTIONS

Depression/Mental Health

Studies have demonstrated that patients who have depressive disorders have worse outcomes and are prone to adverse events following orthopedic surgery compared with controls.[10–12] Specifically in TSA, Swiggett and colleagues found patients who have depressive disorders undergoing primary TSA have an increased in-hospital LOS, in addition to greater odds of readmissions, medical complications, and implant-related complications.[11] This was backed by Bot and colleagues who also noted that depression significantly increased the odds of adverse events following shoulder arthroplasty, including medical complications such as postoperative anemia, pulmonary insufficiency, and need for transfusions of blood products.[10] Due to these findings, it may be prudent to include a depression screening tool in preoperative assessments before TSA. If positive, patients should be given resources for counseling or psychiatric consult before surgery.

Smoking Cessation

Literature has shown that smoking cessation interventions before surgery lead to reductions in adverse surgical outcomes, including wound, pulmonary, and overall complications.[16] In TSA literature specifically, Hatta and colleagues examined 1834 shoulders in 1614 patients and found smokers had lower periprosthetic infection-free survival rates and overall complication-free survival rates than nonsmokers. Additionally, they found improved outcomes in those who quit smoking preoperatively when compared with those who continued to smoke, emphasizing the need for preoperative smoking-cessation programs.[57]

In an analysis by Greenberg and colleagues, the authors postulate that smoking is the most important risk factor for postoperative complications after surgery.[16] In light of current literature, smoking status should be routinely identified, documented, and treated preoperatively when considering TSA[57,58] targeting a quit date of at least 8 weeks before surgery, clinicians can reduce perioperative smoking rates and postoperative complication rates.[16] Surgeons can refer patients to their primary care physician or an addiction medicine specialist for pharmacologic help in the smoking cessation process. Overall, given the substantial benefits of quitting, a preoperative smoking-cessation program should be offered to all patients considering TSA.

Preoperative Opioid Use

Literature has demonstrated that preoperative opioid use in TSA leads to inferior clinical outcome scores.[59,60] Furthermore, in a large database study, Wilson and colleagues found that opioid use before TSA is common and is also associated with increased postoperative complications, health-care utilization, revision surgery, and costs. They found that this risk is dose-dependent; therefore, cessation efforts should be made before surgery in order to optimize outcomes.[61] A frank discussion with patients before surgery can lead to a mutually agreed on plan to reduce opioid consumption before TSA surgery. Literature in lower extremity orthopedic procedures found a 5-minute preoperative opioid weaning counseling session resulted in a statistically significant reduction in postoperative opioid consumption.[62] In regard to upper extremity orthopedic procedures, a randomized clinical trial was performed by Syed and colleagues who demonstrated that a preoperative narcotics education program resulted in significantly less consumption of narcotics at 3-month follow-up after shoulder arthroscopic rotator cuff repair.[63] It was also shown in this study that patients that received this education were significantly more likely to discontinue narcotic use by end of follow-up and that this effect was especially pronounced in patients with preoperative narcotic use. In a 2-year follow-up study of this program, it was further demonstrated that this preoperative opiate education program has long-term effects of reducing opiate dependence.[64] These findings highlight both the ease with which a time-efficient intervention can be incorporated into preoperative surgical optimization and the significant impact this can have on patient narcotic use and opiate dependence.

SUMMARY

In summary, the rate of TSA has dramatically increased during recent decades and will continue to increase during coming years. With this large increase in total volume of shoulder arthroplasty comes increased numbers of complications. The risk of many complications can be significantly reduced with appropriate preoperative medical optimization of comorbid conditions. It is the responsibility of the operating surgeon to understand these conditions, appropriately screen patients for them, and ensure that they are treated accordingly before surgery. Most of these conditions can be screened for with simple laboratory or clinical tests and treated with either pharmacologic means or lifestyle modification. Literature has consistently demonstrated that optimizing these conditions preoperatively in the patient undergoing TSA serve to decrease the risk of complications, improve clinical outcomes, and reduce overall health-care costs. However, despite this evidence, further research should be performed to clarify best practice for optimization of these comorbidities in TSA specifically in order to establish formative guidelines in this patient population and to identify patient-specific risk profiles for those undergoing TSA.

CLINICS CARE POINTS

- Diabetes is associated with higher postoperative complications in general and higher medical costs in the patient undergoing TSA due to increased nonhome discharge, length of stay (LOS), and readmissions. Regular preoperative screening for diabetes should be conducted with a goal HgbA1c of less than 7.5%.
- Cardiac conditions are among the most important independent risk factors for complication and mortality. All patients with a cardiac history or age older than 65 years should undergo regular preoperative screening, which includes EKG. Preop BNP is an additional laboratory value that can be considered to better risk stratify and optimize cardiac risk. Patients should be appropriately referred if further intervention is needed.
- Anemia is defined as hemoglobin level less than 120 g/L in women and less than 130 g/L in men. Anemia in the patient undergoing TSA is associated with increased risk for complication, length of hospital stay, readmission rate, and reoperation rate. Regular preoperative screening should be conducted to mitigate this risk. One can also consider obtaining a ferritin level as iron deficiency anemia is the most common form.
- Appropriate management of anticoagulation is another important strategy for medical optimization. Ideally, a goal international normalized ratio of less than 1.3 to 1.4 should be achieved to minimize the risk of complication. Specific management such as the decision to hold anticoagulation, length of time to hold preoperatively, or need for bridging medication is specific to the anticoagulation and patient's risk factors. Referral to vascular medicine or cardiology may be necessary.
- Malnutrition is defined as albumin less than 3.5 g/dL. In general, malnutrition is associated with worse postoperative outcomes including the risk of complications, delayed recovery, poor wound healing, increased hospital LOS, and infection. It has not yet been fully elucidated if preoperative nutritional supplementation improves outcomes in TSA specifically.
- Vitamin D deficiency is defined as 25-hydroxyvitamin D level less than 32 ng/mL. In the setting of TSA, vitamin D deficiency has been shown to be associated with increased risk of revision. A 25-hydroxyvitamin D level should be obtained as part of standard preoperative screening and treated as needed.
- Mental illness, most notably depression, is associated with increased LOS, rate of readmission, medical complications, and implant-related complications in the setting of TSA. Screening for depression or other mental illness should be conducted preoperatively and managed accordingly before surgery.
- Smoking is associated with higher postoperative infection rate and other complication after TSA. Smoking status should be part of regular screening and treated as necessary with either cessation program or referral to addiction specialist. Cessation at least 8 weeks before surgery has been shown to reduce complications.
- Preoperative opiate use is associated with worse clinical outcomes scores, postoperative complications, health-care utilization, revision surgery, and costs after TSA. Effort should be made to safely reduce opiate use before TSA with either appropriate counseling from treating surgeon, referral to specialist, or enrollment in specialized program.

DECLARATION OF INTERESTS

The authors have nothing to disclose.

REFERENCES

1. Anthony CA, Westermann RW, Gao Y, et al. What are risk factors for 30-day morbidity and transfusion in total shoulder arthroplasty? a review of 1922 cases clinical orthopaedics and related research. Clin Orthop Relat Res 1999;473:2099–105.
2. Wagner ER, Farley KX, Higgins MB, et al. The incidence of shoulder arthroplasty: rise and future projections compared with hip and knee arthroplasty.

J Shoulder Elbow Surg [Internet] 2020. https://doi.org/10.1016/j.jse.2020.03.049.
3. Aldinger PR, Raiss P, Rickert M, et al. Complications in shoulder arthroplasty: an analysis of 485 cases. Int Orthop 2010;34:517–24.
4. Traven SA, Mcgurk KM, Reeves RA, et al. Modified frailty index predicts medical complications, length of stay, readmission, and mortality following total shoulder arthroplasty. J Shoulder Elbow Surg 2019. Available at: www.elsevier.com/locate/ymse.
5. Carli F, Baldini G. From preoperative assessment to preoperative optimization of frail older patiens. Eur J Surg Oncol 2021. https://doi.org/10.1016/j.ejso.2020.06.011.
6. Myatra S, Divatia J v, Jibhkate B, et al. Preoperative assessment and optimization in periampullary and pancreatic cancer. Indian J Cancer 2011;48(1): 86–93. Available at: https://www.indianjcancer.com/printarticle.asp?issn=0019-509X;year=2011;volume=48;issue=1;spage=86;epage=93;aulast=Myatra.
7. Cole WW, Familia M, Miskimin C, et al. Preoperative optimization and tips to avoiding surgical complications before the incision. Sports Med Arthrosc Rev 2022;30(1):2–9. Available at: www.sportsmedarthro.com.
8. Dlott CC, Moore A, Nelson C, et al. Preoperative risk factor optimization lowers hospital length of stay and postoperative emergency department visits in primary total hip and knee arthroplasty patients. J Arthroplasty 2020. https://doi.org/10.1016/j.arth.2020.01.083.
9. Feely MA, Scott Collins C, Daniels PR, et al. Preoperative testing before noncardiac surgery: Guidelines and Recommendations. Am Fam Physician [Internet] 2013;87(6):414–8. Available at: www.aafp.org/afp.
10. Bot AGJ, Menendez ME, Neuhaus V, et al. The influence of psychiatric comorbidity on perioperative outcomes after shoulder arthroplasty. J Shoulder Elbow Surg 2014;23:519–27.
11. Swiggett SJ, Vakharia AM, Ehiorobo JO, et al. Impact of depressive disorders on primary total shoulder arthroplasties: a matched control analysis of 113,648 Medicare patients. Shoulder Elbow 2021;13(2):181–7.
12. Gold HT, Slover JD, Joo L, et al. Association of depression with 90-day hospital readmission after total joint arthroplasty. J Arthroplasty 2016;31: 2385–8. Available at:.
13. Sahoo S, Derwin KA, Zajichek A, et al, Cleveland Clinic Shoulder Group. Associations of preoperative patient mental health status and sociodemographic and clinical characteristics with baseline pain, function, and satisfaction in patients undergoing primary shoulder arthroplasty. J Shoulder Elbow Surg 2021 [cited 2022 Oct 29];30:212–24. Available at: www.elsevier.com/locate/ymse.
14. Sridharan MJ, Everhart JS, Frantz TL, et al. High prevalence of outpatient falls following elective shoulder arthroplasty. J Shoulder Elbow Surg [Internet 2020 [cited 2022 Nov 20];29:699–706.
15. Schairer WW, Zhang AL, Feeley BT. Hospital readmissions after primary shoulder arthroplasty. J Shoulder Elbow Surg 2014 [cited 2022 Oct 21];23:1349–55.
16. Greenberg JA, Zwiep TM, Sadek J, et al. Clinical practice guideline: evidence, recommendations and algorithm for the preoperative optimization of anemia, hyperglycemia and smoking. Can J Surg 2021;64(5):e491–509.
17. Frisch A, Chandra P, Smiley D, et al. Prevalence and clinical outcome of hyperglycemia in the perioperative period in noncardiac surgery. Diabetes Care 2010 [cited 2022 Oct 21];33(8):1783–8. Available from: http://creativecommons.
18. Mahure S, Mollon B, Quien M, et al. Impact of diabetes on perioperative complications in patients undergoing elective total shoulder arthroplasty. Bull Hosp Jt Dis 2013;75(3):173–9.
19. Scott KL, Chung AS, Makovicka JL, et al. Ninety-day readmissions following reverse total shoulder arthroplasty. JSES Open Access 2019;3:54–8 [cited 2022 Oct 21].
20. American Diabetes Association. 2. Classification and diagnosis of diabetes: standards of medical care in diabetes — 2018. Diabetes Care [Internet] 2018;41(Supplement 1): S13–27[cited 2022 Oct 21].
21. Kavin M, Yayac M, Grosso MJ, et al. preoperative hemoglobin A1c >7.5 is associated with increased bundled payment costs in total hip and knee arthroplasties. J Am Acad Orthop Surg 2021; 29(22):970–6.
22. Cancienne JM, Brockmeier SF, Werner BC. Association of perioperative glycemic control with deep postoperative infection after shoulder arthroplasty in patients with diabetes. J Am Acad Orthop Surg 2018;26(11):e238–45.
23. Mcelvany MD, Chan PH, Prentice HA, et al. Diabetes disease severity was not associated with risk of deep infection or revision after shoulder arthroplasty. Clin Orthop Relat Res 2019;477:1358–69.
24. Koh J, Galvin JW, Sing DC, et al. Thirty-day complications and readmission rates in elderly patients after shoulder arthroplasty. J Am Acad Orthop Surg Glob Res Rev 2018;2(11).
25. Waterman BR, Dunn JC, Bader J, et al. Thirty-day morbidity and mortality after elective total shoulder arthroplasty: patient-based and surgical risk factors. J Shoulder Elbow Surg 2015;24:24–30 [cited 2022 Oct 21].
26. Farng E, Zingmond D, Krenek L, et al. Factors predicting complication rates after primary shoulder

arthroplasty. J Shoulder Elbow Surg 2011 [cited 2022 Oct 21];20:557–63. Available at: www.elsevier.com/locate/ymse.

27. Correll DJ, Hepner DL, Chang C, et al. Preoperative electrocardiograms: patient factors predictive of abnormalities. Anesthesiology [Internet] 2009 [cited 2022 Oct 29];110(6):1217–22. Available at: www.anesthesiology.org.
28. Breidthardt T, Kindler CH, Schindler C, et al. B-type natriuretic peptide in patients undergoing orthopaedic surgery: A prospective cohort study. Eur J Anaesthesiol 2010;27(8):690–5.
29. Fox HM, Best MJ, Mikula JD, et al. Short-term complications and readmission following total shoulder arthroplasty: A national database study. Archives of Bone and Joint Surgery 2021;9(3): 323–9.
30. World Health Organization. The global prevalence of anaemia in 2011 [Internet]. Geneva. 2015. Available at. www.who.int.
31. Hollowell JG, Assendelft OW, Gunter EW, et al. Hematological and iron-related analytes — reference data for persons aged 1 year and over: United States, 1988–94. Vital and Health Statistics 2005; 11(247):1–156.
32. Alexander DP, Frew N. Preoperative optimisation of anaemia for primary total hip arthroplasty: a systematic review. Hip Int 2017;27(6):515–22.
33. Dix B, Grant-McDonald L, Catanzariti A, et al. Preoperative anemia in hindfoot and ankle arthrodesis. Foot Ankle Spec 2017;10(2):109–15.
34. Doan MK, Pollock JR, Moore ML, et al. Increasing severity of anemia is associated with poorer 30-day outcomes for total shoulder arthroplasty. JSES Int [Internet] 2021. https://doi.org/10.1016/j.jseint.2021.02.001 [cited 2022 Oct 21];5:360–4. Available at:.
35. Camaschella C. Iron-Deficiency Anemia. Longo DL, editor. New England Journal of medicine. 2015;372(19):1832–1843. Available at: http://www.nejm.org/doi/10.1056/NEJMra1401038
36. O'Donnell M, Kearon C. Perioperative management of oral anticoagulation. Cardiol Clin 2008;26: 299–309.
37. Thakur NA, Czerwein JK, Butera JN, et al. Perioperative management of chronic anticoagulation in orthopaedic surgery. J Am Acad Orthop Surg 2010; 18(12):729–38.
38. Ashkenazi I, Schermann H, Gold · Aviram, et al. Is continuation of anti-platelet treatment safe for elective total hip arthroplasty patients? Arch Orthop Trauma Surg 2020. https://doi.org/10.1007/s00402-020-03629-7 [cited 2022 Oct 21];140:2101–7. Available at:.
39. Servin F. Low-dose aspirin and clopidogrel: how to act in patients scheduled for day surgery. Curr Opin Anaesthesiol 2007;20:531–4.
40. Rogers TH, Labott JR, Austin DC, et al. Perioperative clopidogrel (Plavix) continuation in shoulder arthroplasty: approach cautiously. JSES Int [Internet] 2022. https://doi.org/10.1016/j.jseint.2022.01.008 [cited 2022 Oct 29];6:406–12. Available at:.
41. Flamant EM, Goltz DE, Burnett RA, et al. Malnutrition in elective shoulder arthroplasty: a multi-institutional retrospective study of preoperative albumin and adverse outcomes. J Shoulder Elbow Surg 2021;30:2491–7 [cited 2022 Oct 21].
42. Black CS, Goltz DE, Ryan SP, et al. The role of malnutrition in ninety-day outcomes after total joint arthroplasty. J Arthroplasty 2019;34:2594–600 [cited 2022 Oct 21].
43. Padegimas EM, Maltenfort M, Ramsey ML, et al. Periprosthetic shoulder infection in the United States: incidence and economic burden. J Shoulder Elbow Surg 2015;24:741–6 [cited 2022 Nov 16].
44. Garcia GH, Fu MC, Dines DM, et al. Malnutrition: a marker for increased complications, mortality, and length of stay after total shoulder arthroplasty. J Shoulder Elbow Surg 2016;25:193–200 [cited 2022 Nov 16].
45. Gillis C, Wischmeyer PE. Pre-operative nutrition and the elective surgical patient: why, how and what? Anaesthesia 2019 [cited 2022 Oct 21];74(Suppl. 1):27–35. Available at: https://associationofanaesthetists-publications.onlinelibrary.wiley.com/doi/10.1111/anae.14506.
46. Zhong JX, Kang Mm K, Shu XL. Effect of nutritional support on clinical outcomes in perioperative malnourished patients: a meta-analysis. Asia Pac J Clin Nutr 2015 [cited 2022 Oct 21];24(3):367–78. Available at: http://www.cnki.net/.
47. Ng M, Fleming TB, Robinson MB, et al. Global, regional, and national prevalence of overweight and obesity in children and adults during 1980-2013: a systematic analysis for the Global Burden of Disease Study. 2013. 2014 [cited 2022 Nov 17];384. Available at: www.thelancet.com.
48. Davis AM, Wood AM, Keenan ACM, et al. Does body mass index affect clinical outcome post-operatively and at five years after primary unilateral total hip replacement performed for osteoarthritis? A Multivariate Analysis of Prospective Date. J Bone Joint Surg 2011;93-B(9):1178–82.
49. Dowsey MM, Choong PFM. Obese diabetic patients are at substantial risk for deep infection after primary TKA. Clin Orthop Relat Res 2009;467:1577–81.
50. Friedman RJ, Hess S, Berkowitz SD, et al. Complication rates after hip or knee arthroplasty in morbidly obese patients. Clin Orthop Relat Res 2013;471:3358–66.
51. Wagner ER, Houdek MT, Schleck C, et al. Increasing body mass index is associated with

worse outcomes after shoulder arthroplasty. Journal of Bone and Joint Surgery - American 2017; 99-A(11):929–37.
52. Smith JM, Cancienne JM, Brockmeier SF, et al. Vitamin D deficiency and total shoulder arthroplasty complications. Shoulder Elbow 2021; 13(1):99–105. Available at: http://www.pearldi-.
53. Otto RJ, Virani NA, Levy JC, et al. Scapular fractures after reverse shoulder arthroplasty: evaluation of risk factors and the reliability of a proposed classification. J Shoulder Elbow Surg [Internet 2013;22: 1514–21 [cited 2022 Oct 29].
54. Lau SC, Large R. Acromial fracture after reverse total shoulder arthroplasty: a systematic review. Shoulder Elbow 2020;12(6):375–89.
55. Ko S, Chae S, Choi W, et al. The effectiveness of vitamin D supplementation in functional outcome and quality of life (QoL) of lumbar spinal stenosis (LSS) requiring surgery. J Orthop Surg Res [Internet 2020 [cited 2022 Oct 21];15:117. Available at: http://creativecommons.org/licenses/by/4.0/TheCreativeCommonsPublicDomainDedicationwaiver.
56. Sprague S, Slobogean GP, Cowley A. Vitamin D use and health outcomes after surgery for hip fracture. FAITH Investigators 2017;40(5):e868–75.
57. Hatta T, Werthel JD, Wagner ER, et al. Effect of smoking on complications following primary shoulder arthroplasty. J Shoulder Elbow Surg 2017. https://doi.org/10.1016/j.jse.2016.09.011 [cited 2022 Oct 21];26:1–6. Available at:.
58. Althoff AD, Reeves RA, Traven SA, et al. Smoking is associated with increased surgical complications following total shoulder arthroplasty: an analysis of 14,465 patients. J Shoulder Elbow Surg 2020 [cited 2022 Oct 21];29:491–6. Available at: www.elsevier.com/locate/ymse.
59. Thompson KM, Hallock JD, Smith RA, et al. Preoperative narcotic use and inferior outcomes after anatomic total shoulder arthroplasty: a clinical and radiographic analysis. J Am Acad Orthop Surg 2019; 27(5):177–82.
60. Nadarajah V, Meredith SJ, Jauregui JJ, et al. Preoperative opioid use in patients undergoing shoulder surgery. Shoulder Elbow 2021;13(3):248–59.
61. Wilson JM, Farley KX, Gottschalk MB, et al. Preoperative opioid use is an independent risk factor for complication, revision, and increased health care utilization following primary total shoulder arthroplasty. J Shoulder Elbow Surg 2021;30(5):1025–33.
62. Paskey T, Vincent S, Critchlow E, et al. Prospective randomized study evaluating the effects of preoperative opioid counseling on postoperative opioid use after outpatient lower extremity orthopaedic surgery. J Surg Orthop Adv 2021;30(1):2–6.
63. Ali Syed UM, Aleem AW, Wowkanech C, et al. Neer Award 2018: the effect of preoperative education on opioid consumption in patients undergoing arthroscopic rotator cuff repair: a prospective, randomized clinical trial. J Shoulder Elbow Surg 2018; 27:962–7 [cited 2022 Nov 17].
64. Cheesman Q, Defrance M, Stenson J, et al. The effect of preoperative education on opioid consumption in patients undergoing arthroscopic rotator cuff repair: a prospective, randomized clinical trial - 2-year follow-up. J Shoulder Elbow Surg 2020; 29:1743–50 [cited 2022 Nov 17].

Modifiable and Nonmodifiable Risk Factors Associated with the Development of Recurrent Rotator Cuff Tears

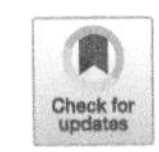

Brendan M. Patterson, MD, MPH*,
Maria F. Bozoghlian, MD

KEYWORDS

• Rotator cuff retear • Surgical repair • Risk factors

KEY POINTS

- There are nonmodifiable and modifiable risk factors for retear following rotator cuff repair surgery.
- Most of the nonmodifiable risk factors are consistent among the literature and have been thoroughly studied, such as age, tear size, muscular atrophy, and fatty infiltration.
- There are other nonmodifiable risk factors that remain controversial in the current literature.
- When considering modifiable risk factors for retear after surgical repair, there are some consistencies and discrepancies in the literature. Nevertheless, optimizing modifiable risk factors, when possible, has the potential to decrease retear following rotator cuff repair surgery.

INTRODUCTION

Rotator cuff tears are one of the most common causes of shoulder pain and disability.[1,2] Several authors have investigated the prevalence of rotator cuff tears in cadaveric and population-based studies.[1,3,4] It is well known that the prevalence of rotator cuff disease increases with age,[3] but there are other important risk factors associated with this common shoulder condition.[1] The progression and natural history of degenerative rotator cuff tears has been previously studied,[2] and surgeons must account for several factors when considering surgical versus nonsurgical treatment options.

Nonsurgical treatment, including physical therapy, various types of injections, and activity modification, is effective for many patients with symptomatic rotator cuff tears.[5] Surgical repair of rotator cuff tears is a widely used treatment option for symptomatic rotator cuff tears, especially in the acute setting, or when conservative treatment has failed. Nevertheless, recurrent tears after surgical repair are a frequently observed complication,[6] and the incidence of retears remains a concern among surgeons, regardless of the surgical technique performed. Prospective studies have shown failure rates ranging from 15% to 30% after arthroscopic rotator cuff repair,[7–9] and the published literature shows significant heterogeneity in the retear rates.[10]

Several risk factors have been studied in relation to the probability of recurrent rotator cuff tear after surgical repair. Although some risk factors are well defined in the available literature, others remain under discussion, and many published articles show controversial results. This

Department of Orthopedics and Rehabilitation, University of Iowa, 200 Hawkins Drive, Iowa City, IA 52242, USA
* Corresponding author.
E-mail address: brendan-patterson@uiowa.edu

Orthop Clin N Am 54 (2023) 319–326
https://doi.org/10.1016/j.ocl.2023.02.009

article reviews the current literature regarding modifiable and nonmodifiable risk factors for rotator cuff retear after surgical repair.

NONMODIFIABLE RISK FACTORS

Patient Age

Many studies have investigated the relationship between patient age and rotator cuff retear following surgical repair.[7,11–15] Park and colleagues[12] studied prognostic factors affecting rotator cuff healing in small to medium size tears and found that retear rate after arthroscopic repair was significantly higher in patients older than 69 years of age. Furthermore, two recent systematic reviews conducted to evaluate the risk of cuff retear after surgery found that age was significantly associated with a higher risk of retear, especially for those patients greater than 60 years of age.[11,14] A retrospective cohort study conducted by Lee and colleagues[13] involving 693 patients, showed a significant difference in patient age in the retear group when compared with patients with a healed repair. The mean age in the retear group was 64.6 years of age, whereas the mean age in the intact group was 59.1 years of age ($P < .0001$). Additionally, their multivariate analysis showed that patient age was an independent risk factor for retear. Similarly, Le and colleagues[16] found a positive correlation between increased age and risk of rotator cuff retear. Le and colleagues[16] found that as the patient age increased so did the risk of retear. A systematic review and meta-analysis conducted by Khazzam and colleagues[10] showed that the risk of retear doubled from 15% at age 50 to 31% at age 70. The results from the previously mentioned studies all demonstrate that patient age remains one of the most important independent risk factors associated with retear following rotator cuff repair.

Tear Size and Retraction

In addition to patient age, tear size and the amount of tendon retraction are also important factors to consider preoperatively, not only for surgical decision making, but also as potential risk factors for decreased healing capacity following rotator cuff repair. Most of the published literature has found tear size and retraction to be directly related to the probability of rotator cuff retear following surgical repair.[7,11–14,17–23] Le and colleagues,[16] in their retrospective cohort study of 1000 patients undergoing rotator cuff repair, assessed the association of tear size and retear following rotator cuff repair. They specifically investigated tear dimensions in the anteroposterior and mediolateral planes. Their results showed that preoperative tear length and tear size area were significantly larger in the retear group, and that increased anteroposterior tear length and increased tear size area had the greatest statistical correlation with retear following surgical repair.[16] Park and colleagues[12] also found tear size to be an independent prognostic factor for cuff healing. Furthermore, they determined a critical tear size value of 2 cm for successful rotator cuff healing following repair. A more recent systematic review and meta-analysis conducted to define the incidence of rotator cuff retear after surgical repair, found tear size to be significantly associated with retear rate in 11 of the 31 studies included for analysis.[14]

In addition to tear size, many authors have studied rotator cuff tendon retraction and its influence on healing following repair. Tashjian and colleagues[21] studied the position of the musculotendinous junction (MTJ) in relation to the glenoid face on preoperative MRIs and found that a more medialized MTJ position preoperatively had a lower rate of healing. They also found that the preoperative distance of the MTJ to the glenoid face was significantly correlated with the preoperative sagittal tear size.[21] Other studies have also found retraction and distance of MTJ to the glenoid to be significantly related with the retear rate after arthroscopic repair, with values of retraction of 22.2 mm of tendon retraction to be highly predictive of retear.[11,23]

Fatty Infiltration and Muscular Atrophy

Several authors have studied the relationship between fatty degeneration of the rotator cuff and healing capacity following repair. Goutallier classification has been expanded from its original use and description in computed tomography scans now to MRI.[24,25] The Goutallier classification is widely cited in many articles that investigate the relationship between fatty infiltration of the rotator cuff and the probability of retear after surgical repair.[26] A retrospective review of 196 arthroscopic cuff repairs conducted by Uzun and colleagues[17] found that advanced grade of preoperative Goutallier fatty infiltration was significantly related to a higher probability of retear. Furthermore, a meta-analysis performed by Zhao and colleagues[11] showed that fatty infiltration of the subscapularis and infraspinatus were risk factors for rotator cuff retear, regardless of the Goutallier grade. Increased fatty infiltration, defined as Goutallier grade greater than 2, has been assessed as an independent risk factor for retear by several authors (**Fig. 1**).[13,19,20]

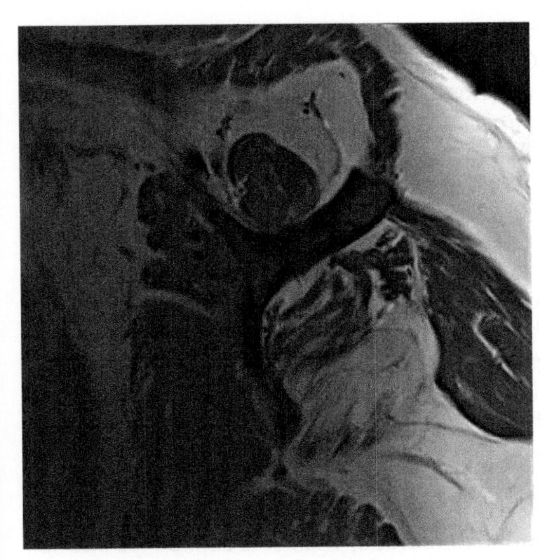

Fig. 1. Sagittal T1 MRI demonstrating preserved rotator cuff muscle of the subscapularis with advanced muscular atrophy of the infraspinatus and teres minor musculature.

Jeong and colleagues[27] evaluated fatty infiltration of the infraspinatus and subscapularis and atrophy and occupation ratio of the supraspinatus. They defined occupation ratio as the ratio between the cross-sectional area of the supraspinatus muscle and the supraspinatus fossa in the scapular Y-view of MRI. They found supraspinatus atrophy and infraspinatus fatty infiltration to be independent risk factors for retear.[27] Occupation ratio of the supraspinatus was significantly lower in the retear group, but there was no difference in subscapularis fatty infiltration between groups. In addition, in their predictive models they established cutoff values of infraspinatus fatty infiltration and supraspinatus occupation ratio to predict the possibility of retear. Fatty infiltration of the infraspinatus of grade 2 or higher, or occupation ratio of the supraspinatus less than 43% were associated with a higher possibility of retear.[27] Similar results were found by Kim and colleagues[23] in their retrospective cohort study of 180 patients with medium to large rotator cuff tears. In addition to tear size and patient age, muscular atrophy and fatty infiltration of the rotator cuff musculature is an important risk factor for rotator cuff retear following repair.

Anatomic Factors: Critical Shoulder Angle and Acromiohumeral Interval

Certain anatomic factors, such as the critical shoulder angle (CSA) and acromiohumeral interval (AHI), have also been studied as potential factors contributing to the probability of rotator cuff retear after surgical repair. The published literature has controversial results regarding the influence of CSA and AHI on the development of recurrent rotator cuff tears. CSA is defined as the angle created by a line connecting the superior and inferior margins of the glenoid, and an intersecting line drawn from the inferior margin of the glenoid to the most lateral border of the acromion (Fig. 2). AHI is defined as the distance between the lower margin of the acromion and the upper margin of the humeral head, in anteroposterior radiographs (Fig. 3). Some authors have demonstrated a significant relationship between CSA and retear rate,[11,18,28,29] whereas others have found no statistically significant relationship.[17,27,30] Garcia and colleagues[28] performed a retrospective review of 76 patients undergoing arthroscopic rotator cuff repair and postoperative ultrasound to evaluate integrity of repair. They found that patients with no signs of a retear had a significantly lower CSA compared with patients with a postoperative full-thickness retear. Furthermore, they established an odds ratio of having a full-thickness retear of 14.8 with a CSA greater than 38°.[28] Liu and colleagues[29] performed a systematic review with meta-analysis to determine the correlation between increased CSA and retear rates following arthroscopic rotator cuff repair. Their analysis showed an association between increased CSA and risk of cuff retear. Conversely, Como and colleagues[30] performed a retrospective review of 164 patients that underwent arthroscopic

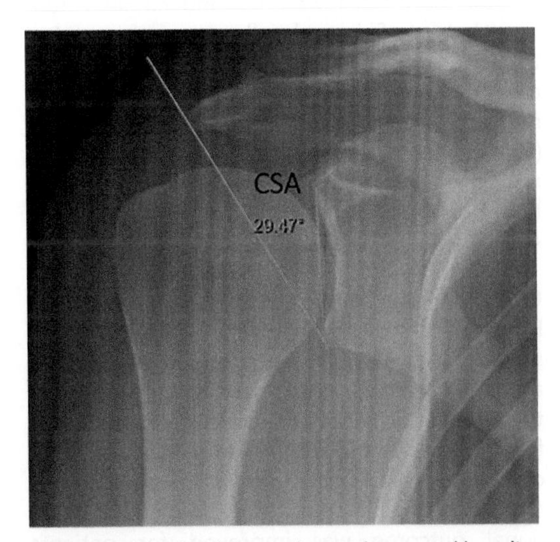

Fig. 2. Critical shoulder angle. Angle created by a line connecting the superior and inferior margins of the glenoid, and an intersecting line drawn from the inferior margin of the glenoid to the most lateral border of the acromion.

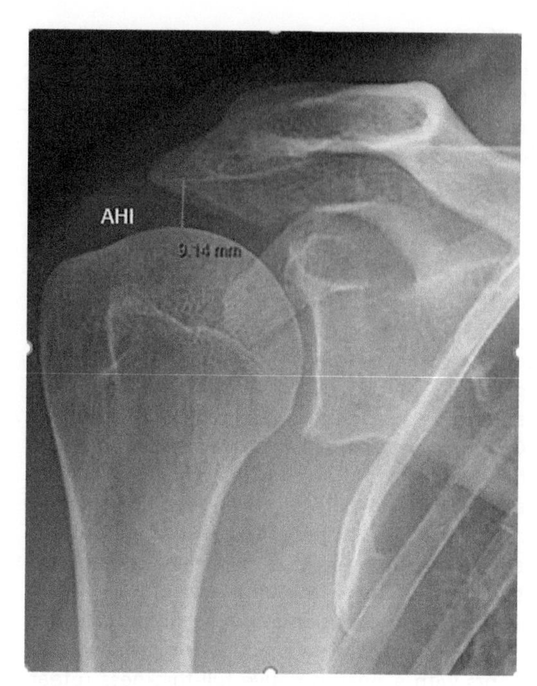

Fig. 3. Acromiohumeral interval. Distance between the lower margin of the acromion and the upper margin of the humeral head.

rotator cuff repair in which CSA was measured for all patients. The average CSA in the nonretear group was 32.3° ± 4.7°, whereas the average CSA in the retear group was 31.2° ± 4.5°, showing no association.[30] Similar conflicting results have been published regarding AHI. Some authors have found a correlation between lower AHI and higher retear rate.[11,23,27,31] Shin and colleagues[31] found AHI to be an independent risk factor for rotator cuff retear, with results showing that risk of retear of supraspinatus decreased 0.512 times (95% confidence interval, 0.33–0.794) for every millimeter of increased AHI. Contrarily, other authors found no significant relationship between AHI and risk of retear.[17,19]

Chronicity and Time to Surgery

Duration of symptoms, and prolonged time to surgery, have been investigated in many studies as potential risk factors for recurrent rotator cuff tears. Gutman and colleagues[32] investigated functional outcomes following early versus delayed surgical management of acute traumatic rotator cuff tears. They found that functional outcome was improved for patients undergoing surgery within 4 months of sustaining an acute rotator cuff tear. Although this study did show functional improvements with early surgery compared with delayed surgery, retear rates were not assessed in this cohort. Other authors have investigated chronicity of symptoms and subsequent retear rate following surgical treatment of rotator cuff tears. Many of these studies have shown that an increased time from symptom onset to surgery is significantly correlated with a higher retear rate.[11,17,33] A database study that queried Humana claims from 2007 to 2016 found an association between delayed rotator cuff repair and revision surgery because of retear. They established three timepoints for initial surgical repair as: (1) early repair within 6 weeks of diagnosis, (2) routine repair between 6 weeks and 12 months after diagnosis, and (3) delayed repair more than 12 months after diagnosis. Results showed an increased odds of revision surgery in the delayed repair group (odds ratio, 1.97; 95% confidence interval, 1.16–3.21; $P = .009$).[33]

Conversely, other authors found no association between prolonged time to surgery and surgical failure or retear rate.[7,34] Finger and colleagues[34] performed a retrospective cohort study of patients with degenerative rotator cuff tears who underwent surgical repair either before 12 months of symptoms onset (early surgery) or after 12 months of symptoms onset (delayed surgery). There were no significant differences found in retear rates or failure rates between the two cohorts. Similar results were found by Le and colleagues[16] in their retrospective cohort study of 1000 patients; although symptom duration time was longer in the retear group (25.4 vs 21.9 months), the difference as compared with the patients with an intact rotator cuff repair was not statistically significant.

MODIFIABLE RISK FACTORS

Diabetes Mellitus

Uncontrolled hyperglycemia can have a detrimental impact on health caused by multisystemic complications. Long-term uncontrolled diabetes can generate damage in several organs, such as kidney and retina, and can also lead to musculoskeletal and tissue-repair disorders. In regards to surgical procedures, the association with uncontrolled hyperglycemia and increased risk of infection is well known.[35] However, the effect of diabetes on tendon healing, specifically after arthroscopic repair of the rotator cuff, is still controversial. Cho and colleagues[36] conducted a retrospective review of 335 shoulders that underwent arthroscopic rotator cuff repair, with the objective to compare clinical and structural outcomes in patients with and without diabetes. Comparison of preoperative global fatty degeneration index, muscle atrophy, and tear size (among other factors) did not show significant differences between the patients with and without diabetes. All shoulders underwent an MRI, at least 6 months after surgery, and a higher retear rate was found between the diabetic cohort compared with the nondiabetic cohort (35.9% vs 14.4%, respectively; $P < .001$).[36] Furthermore, the retear rates according to levels of hemoglobin A_{1c} (HbA_{1c}) were measured. In patients with uncontrolled diabetes ($HbA_{1c} \geq 7\%$) the retear rate was 43.2%, whereas in patients with controlled diabetes ($HbA_{1c} < 7\%$), the retear rate was 25.9% ($P < .001$).[36] In addition to the previously noted findings from Cho and colleagues,[36] a meta-analysis conducted by Zhao and colleagues[11] reported on the impact of diabetes and rotator cuff healing. This meta-analysis demonstrated that diabetes was a risk factor for retear after arthroscopic rotator cuff repair. Kim and colleagues[23] found a moderate association between patients with diagnosis of diabetes mellitus and retear rates ($P = .46$), in their multivariate analysis. Uzun and colleagues[17] performed a retrospective review of 196 shoulders to analyze risk factors for rotator cuff retear following arthroscopic repair. They found no association between diabetes and the risk of retear ($P = .432$). Although diabetes mellitus is often included as a comorbidity in many studies in the current literature, the distinction between controlled and uncontrolled diabetes is not always made. Nevertheless, based current data, surgeons should make efforts to optimize levels of HbA_{1c} in patients with diabetes before rotator cuff repair.

Hyperlipidemia and Body Mass Index

Hyperlipidemia has been studied as a potential risk factor for tendon pathology. Various studies performed in animal models have evaluated the impact on hyperlipidemia in the healing properties of the rotator cuff, showing hypercholesterolemia having a deleterious effect on tendon quality.[37] Garcia and colleagues[38] conducted a retrospective review of 85 arthroscopic rotator cuff repairs, with all patients undergoing postoperative ultrasound at 6 months following surgery. In their cohort, 38.8% of patients had hyperlipidemia, and all of them were being treated with statins. The retear rate in the group with hyperlipidemia was 45.5% (partial and full tears), compared with a rate of 11.3% in the nonhyperlipidemia group, with an odds ratio of 6.5 ($P < .001$).[38] Harada and colleagues[18] conducted a retrospective review of 286 patients and found that hyperlipidemia was an independent risk factor for rotator cuff retear. Furthermore, hyperlipidemia was included as a risk factor in their decision tree model for prediction of retear within the groups with a higher risk for retear.[18]

Body mass index (BMI) is usually taken into consideration as a comorbidity in most orthopedic surgical procedures. Elevated BMI has been associated with a higher rate of postoperative complications after arthroscopic repair of rotator cuff tears. Rubenstein and colleagues[39] conducted a database study to assess complication rates after shoulder arthroscopic procedures in relation with patients' BMI values, and found that complication rates were higher in patients with BMI greater than 40 when compared with patients with a BMI less than 40. Furthermore, Gumina and colleagues[40] studied the relationship between BMI and rotator cuff tear size, finding that patients with massive tears had a greater BMI. Nevertheless, regarding tendon healing and retear rate after arthroscopic repair, the results found in literature remain controversial. A case-control study performed by Ersen and colleagues[41] to evaluate retear rate and predictive factors for repair failure in small to medium size rotator cuff tears, reported BMI as an independent predictive factor for repair failure. Their receiver operating characteristic curve analyses established a BMI cutoff value of 28.1, showing that repair failure in patients with BMI greater than 28.1 was significantly higher compared with patients with a BMI less than 28.1 ($P = .001$). Other authors have also found a significant relationship between high BMI and retear rates.[11,23] Conversely, some published literature that analyzed patients' BMI and retear rates, found no significant association. Uzun and colleagues[17] found that even though the median BMI was higher in the retear group, the difference was not statistically significant. Similar results were found by Jeong and colleagues[27] in their case-control study to determine predictive risk factors for retear. Nevertheless, high BMI, especially when surpassing obesity values, is often associated with other metabolic conditions that altogether increase the risk of postoperative complications, and may influence healing rates following rotator cuff repair.

Bone Mineral Density

Bone mineral density (BMD) may also play an important role in rotator cuff repair healing, because secure fixation either through suture anchors or bone tunnels influences the integrity of the repair at time zero following repair. Previous cadaveric studies have established a relationship between BMD and pullout strength of suture anchors.[42,43] Chung and colleagues[44] performed a retrospective cohort study of patients with full thickness rotator cuff tears who underwent arthroscopic repair. They found a retear rate of 9% in patients with BMD greater than −1 (normal BMD), 30.2% in patients with BMD between −2.5 and −1 (osteopenia), and a retear rate of 41.7% in patients with BMD less than −2.5 (osteoporosis). Similar results were found in a meta-analysis performed by Zhao and colleagues[11] to assess risk factors affecting rotator cuff retear. BMD is increased with the use of medications and nonmedication therapies, such as dietary modifications and exercise. As such, this may be a modifiable risk factor to consider optimization for before rotator cuff repair when possible.

Smoking

Smoking has been associated many adverse outcomes following orthopedic procedures, most notably wound, boney, and soft tissue healing issues.[45] Despite these known complications, the available literature shows somewhat conflicting findings in regards to the relationship between smoking and rotator cuff healing following repair. Santiago-Torres and coworkers[46] conducted a systematic review to determine the effects of smoking on soft tissue healing following shoulder surgery. They found five studies evaluating the healing capacity or structural outcomes after repair. One basic science study included in the systematic review showed a delay in tendon to bone healing in relationship with smoking; however, the other four clinical studies had controversial results, with only one study finding a significant negative effect of smoking on tendon healing.[46] Furthermore, other clinical studies have not demonstrated a significant relationship between smoking status and rotator cuff retear rate.[11,17,18] Most studies consider smoking status as a covariate, and literature evaluating only smoking status and controlling for other confounders is limited.

Exercise and Work Level

When assessing postoperative outcomes of rotator cuff repair and postsurgical complications, it is important to consider the type of activities patients desire to return to after surgery. Kwon and colleagues[47] performed a case-control study to determine factors predictive of rotator cuff healing after surgical repair. They classified their cohort according to exercise level in high, medium, and low. The same classification was used for work activity level as heavy manual labor, medium level, and low level (sedentary work). Their multivariate analysis showed level of work activity to be an independent risk factor for healing capability of the rotator cuff.[47] Conversely, other studies have found no relationship on demanding work or high sports activity level with the risk of rotator cuff retear following surgical repair.[11,19] Given the previously noted conflicting results, this topic remains controversial in the literature. Some sports or working activities are well defined and standardized in some studies, whereas in others the distinction between high- and low-impact sports activities or high-/low-level work activities is not clearly standardized, and therefore it can create disparities in the variables measured. At present time there is no consensus in the literature regarding high- or low-impact sport or working activities that may influence rotator cuff retear following surgery.

SUMMARY

Rotator cuff tears are a common cause of pain and disability among patients with shoulder pathology. Nonoperative and operative strategies exist to manage rotator cuff pathology. Although rotator cuff repair is successful for most patients, some patients may experience retear or nonhealing of the rotator cuff after surgery. Several risk factors, modifiable and nonmodifiable, have been associated with an increased retear rate following rotator cuff repair. The literature shows consistency and agreement in regards to many of these risk factors, most notably, patient age and tear size, and rotator cuff muscular atrophy. Other risk factors for retear following rotator cuff repair remain controversial. Nevertheless, it is of great importance for shoulder surgeons to be familiar with the modifiable and nonmodifiable risk factors associated with retear following rotator cuff repair surgery. Knowledge of these risk factors allows surgeons to better advise patients and optimize their chances of success following rotator cuff repair surgery.

CLINICS CARE POINTS

- Increased patient age and increased tear size remain the most consistent and well-studied risk factors for retear following rotator cuff repair.
- Rotator cuff muscular atrophy and fatty infiltration as defined by the Goutallier classification is an important nonmodifiable risk factor when considering retear following rotator cuff repair surgery.

- Other nonmodifiable risk factors for rotator cuff retear following surgery are more controversial including: anatomic factors, such as the critical shoulder angle and acromiohumeral interval; duration of symptoms; and chronicity of injury before repair.
- Modifiable risk factors that can influence retear rates following rotator cuff repair include: diabetes mellitus, hyperlipidemia, body mass index, smoking status, bone mineral density, and activity level.
- Although many of the modifiable risk factors for retear following rotator cuff repair are controversial, it is still advisable to optimize modifiable risk factors when possible, before rotator cuff repair.

DISCLOSURE

The authors have nothing to disclose.

REFERENCES

1. Tashjian RZ. Epidemiology, natural history, and indications for treatment of rotator cuff tears. Clin Sports Med 2012;31(4):589–604.
2. Keener JD, Patterson BM, Orvets N, et al. Degenerative rotator cuff tears: refining surgical indications based on natural history data. J Am Acad Orthop Surg 2019;27(5):156–65.
3. Yamamoto A, Takagishi K, Osawa T, et al. Prevalence and risk factors of a rotator cuff tear in the general population. J Shoulder Elbow Surg 2010;19(1):116–20.
4. Yamaguchi K, Ditsios K, Middleton WD, et al. The demographic and morphological features of rotator cuff disease. A comparison of asymptomatic and symptomatic shoulders. J Bone Joint Surg Am 2006;88(8):1699–704.
5. Kuhn JE, Dunn WR, Sanders R, et al. Effectiveness of physical therapy in treating atraumatic full-thickness rotator cuff tears: a multicenter prospective cohort study. J Shoulder Elbow Surg 2013;22(10):1371–9.
6. Lapner P, Henry P, Athwal GS, et al. Treatment of rotator cuff tears: a systematic review and meta-analysis. J Shoulder Elbow Surg 2022;31(3):e120–9.
7. Boileau P, Brassart N, Watkinson DJ, et al. Arthroscopic repair of full-thickness tears of the supraspinatus: does the tendon really heal? J Bone Joint Surg Am 2005;87(6):1229–40.
8. Barth J, Andrieu K, Fotiadis E, et al. Critical period and risk factors for retear following arthroscopic repair of the rotator cuff. Knee Surg Sports Traumatol Arthrosc 2017;25(7):2196–204.
9. Iannotti JP, Deutsch A, Green A, et al. Time to failure after rotator cuff repair: a prospective imaging study. J Bone Joint Surg Am 2013;95(11):965–71.
10. Khazzam M, Sager B, Box HN, et al. The effect of age on risk of retear after rotator cuff repair: a systematic review and meta-analysis. JSES Int 2020;4(3):625–31.
11. Zhao J, Luo M, Pan J, et al. Risk factors affecting rotator cuff retear after arthroscopic repair: a meta-analysis and systematic review. J Shoulder Elbow Surg 2021;30(11):2660–70.
12. Park JS, Park HJ, Kim SH, et al. Prognostic factors affecting rotator cuff healing after arthroscopic repair in small to medium-sized tears. Am J Sports Med 2015;43(10):2386–92.
13. Lee YS, Jeong JY, Park CD, et al. Evaluation of the risk factors for a rotator cuff retear after repair surgery. Am J Sports Med 2017;45(8):1755–61.
14. Longo UG, Carnevale A, Piergentili I, et al. Retear rates after rotator cuff surgery: a systematic review and meta-analysis. BMC Musculoskelet Disord 2021;22(1):749.
15. Gulotta LV, Nho SJ, Dodson CC, et al. Prospective evaluation of arthroscopic rotator cuff repairs at 5 years: part II–prognostic factors for clinical and radiographic outcomes. J Shoulder Elbow Surg 2011;20(6):941–6.
16. Le BT, Wu XL, Lam PH, et al. Factors predicting rotator cuff retears: an analysis of 1000 consecutive rotator cuff repairs. Am J Sports Med 2014;42(5):1134–42.
17. Uzun E, Misir A, Kizkapan TB, et al. Factors associated with the development of re-tear following arthroscopic rotator cuff repair: a retrospective comparative study. Acta Orthop Traumatol Turc 2021;55(3):213–9.
18. Harada N, Gotoh M, Ishitani E, et al. Combination of risk factors affecting retear after arthroscopic rotator cuff repair: a decision tree analysis. J Shoulder Elbow Surg 2021;30(1):9–15.
19. Lobo-Escolar L, Ramazzini-Castro R, Codina-Grano D, et al. Risk factors for symptomatic retears after arthroscopic repair of full-thickness rotator cuff tears. J Shoulder Elbow Surg 2021;30(1):27–33.
20. Oh JH, Kim SH, Kang JY, et al. Effect of age on functional and structural outcome after rotator cuff repair. Am J Sports Med 2010;38(4):672–8.
21. Tashjian RZ, Hung M, Burks RT, et al. Influence of preoperative musculotendinous junction position on rotator cuff healing using single-row technique. Arthroscopy 2013;29(11):1748–54.
22. Galatz LM, Ball CM, Teefey SA, et al. The outcome and repair integrity of completely arthroscopically repaired large and massive rotator cuff tears. J Bone Joint Surg Am 2004;86(2):219–24.
23. Kim YK, Jung KH, Kim JW, et al. Factors affecting rotator cuff integrity after arthroscopic repair for

medium-sized or larger cuff tears: a retrospective cohort study. J Shoulder Elbow Surg 2018;27(6): 1012–20.
24. Fuchs B, Weishaupt D, Zanetti M, et al. Fatty degeneration of the muscles of the rotator cuff: assessment by computed tomography versus magnetic resonance imaging. J Shoulder Elbow Surg 1999;8(6):599–605.
25. Goutallier D, Bernageau J, Patte D. Assessment of the trophicity of the muscles of the ruptured rotator cuff by CT scan. In: Post M, Morrey B, Hawkins R, editors. Surgery of the shoulder. St. Louis, MO: Mosby; 1990. p. 11–3.
26. Goutallier D, Postel JM, Gleyze P, et al. Influence of cuff muscle fatty degeneration on anatomic and functional outcomes after simple suture of full-thickness tears. J Shoulder Elbow Surg 2003;12(6):550–4.
27. Jeong HY, Kim HJ, Jeon YS, et al. Factors predictive of healing in large rotator cuff tears: is it possible to predict retear preoperatively? Am J Sports Med 2018;46(7):1693–700.
28. Garcia GH, Liu JN, Degen RM, et al. Higher critical shoulder angle increases the risk of retear after rotator cuff repair. J Shoulder Elbow Surg 2017;26(2): 241–5.
29. Liu T, Zhang M, Yang Z, et al. Does the critical shoulder angle influence retear and functional outcome after arthroscopic rotator cuff repair? A systematic review and meta-analysis. Arch Orthop Trauma Surg 2022. https://doi.org/10.1007/s00402-022-04640-w.
30. Como CJ, Hughes JD, Lesniak BP, et al. Critical shoulder angle does not influence retear rate after arthroscopic rotator cuff repair. Knee Surg Sports Traumatol Arthrosc 2021;29(12):3951–5.
31. Shin YK, Ryu KN, Park JS, et al. Predictive factors of retear in patients with repaired rotator cuff tear on shoulder MRI. AJR Am J Roentgenol 2018;210(1): 134–41.
32. Gutman MJ, Joyce CD, Patel MS, et al. Early repair of traumatic rotator cuff tears improves functional outcomes. J Shoulder Elbow Surg 2021;30(11):2475–83.
33. Fu MC, O'Donnell EA, Taylor SA, et al. Delay to arthroscopic rotator cuff repair is associated with increased risk of revision rotator cuff surgery. Orthopedics 2020;43(6):340–4.
34. Finger L, Dunn R, Hughes J, et al. Clinical outcomes secondary to time to surgery for atraumatic rotator cuff tears. J Shoulder Elbow Surg 2022;31(6S):S18–24.
35. Cancienne JM, Brockmeier SF, Werner BC. Association of perioperative glycemic control with deep postoperative infection after shoulder arthroplasty in patients with diabetes. J Am Acad Orthop Surg 2018;26(11):e238–45.
36. Cho NS, Moon SC, Jeon JW, et al. The influence of diabetes mellitus on clinical and structural outcomes after arthroscopic rotator cuff repair. Am J Sports Med 2015;43(4):991–7.
37. Chung SW, Park H, Kwon J, et al. Effect of hypercholesterolemia on fatty infiltration and quality of tendon-to-bone healing in a rabbit model of a chronic rotator cuff tear: electrophysiological, biomechanical, and histological analyses. Am J Sports Med 2016;44(5):1153–64.
38. Garcia GH, Liu JN, Wong A, et al. Hyperlipidemia increases the risk of retear after arthroscopic rotator cuff repair. J Shoulder Elbow Surg 2017;26(12): 2086–90.
39. Rubenstein WJ, Lansdown DA, Feeley BT, et al. The impact of body mass index on complications after shoulder arthroscopy: should surgery eligibility be determined by body mass index cutoffs? Arthroscopy 2019;35(3):741–6.
40. Gumina S, Candela V, Passaretti D, et al. The association between body fat and rotator cuff tear: the influence on rotator cuff tear sizes. J Shoulder Elbow Surg 2014;23(11):1669–74.
41. Ersen A, Sahin K, Albayrak MO. Older age and higher body mass index are independent risk factors for tendon healing in small- to medium-sized rotator cuff tears. Knee Surg Sports Traumatol Arthrosc 2023;31(2):681–90.
42. Yakacki CM, Poukalova M, Guldberg RE, et al. The effect of the trabecular microstructure on the pull-out strength of suture anchors. J Biomech 2010; 43(10):1953–9.
43. Tingart MJ, Apreleva M, Lehtinen J, et al. Anchor design and bone mineral density affect the pull-out strength of suture anchors in rotator cuff repair: which anchors are best to use in patients with low bone quality? Am J Sports Med 2004; 32(6):1466–73.
44. Chung SW, Oh JH, Gong HS, et al. Factors affecting rotator cuff healing after arthroscopic repair: osteoporosis as one of the independent risk factors. Am J Sports Med 2011;39(10):2099–107.
45. Lee JJ, Patel R, Biermann JS, et al. The musculoskeletal effects of cigarette smoking. J Bone Joint Surg Am 2013;95(9):850–9.
46. Santiago-Torres J, Flanigan DC, Butler RB, et al. The effect of smoking on rotator cuff and glenoid labrum surgery: a systematic review. Am J Sports Med 2015;43(3):745–51.
47. Kwon J, Kim SH, Lee YH, et al. The Rotator Cuff Healing Index: a new scoring system to predict rotator cuff healing after surgical repair. Am J Sports Med 2019;47(1):173–80.

Foot and Ankle

Update on Medical Management of Diabetes

Focus on Relevance for Orthopedic Surgeons

Dilasha Katwal, MD, Deirdre James, MD,
Sam Dagogo-Jack, MD, DSc*

KEYWORDS

- Type 1 diabetes • Type 2 diabetes • Microvascular complications • Peripheral vascular disease
- Diabetic foot ulcers • Lower extremity amputations

KEY POINTS

- Diabetes accounts for more than 100,000 lower extremity amputations annually in the United States.
- Peripheral neuropathy, peripheral vascular disease, and foot ulcers are major risk factors for lower extremity amputation in diabetes.
- Optimizing glycemic control and preventing or controlling control of risk factors decrease amputations in people with diabetes.
- Lifestyle interventions, including diet, exercise, weight loss, and smoking cessation, can prevent or delay the progression of microvascular and neurologic complications.
- Adjunctive medications with proven benefits for cardiorenal outcomes increase the chances of preventing diabetes complications.

INTRODUCTION

Diabetes mellitus affects more than 30 million Americans and 537 million people worldwide.[1–3] Type 2 diabetes (T2DM), which accounts for 90% to 95% of the global disease burden, is the major driver of the epidemic.[1,4] Diabetes is the leading cause of kidney disease, lower limb amputation, adult blindness, cardiovascular, and stroke.[1–11] Poorly controlled diabetes is directly related to the development of chronic complications and consequent enormous health care costs.[2,7,12] The economic burden of diabetes-related health expenditure was $327 billion in the United States in 2017 and $966 billion globally in 2021.[2,12]

COMPLICATIONS OF DIABETES

The chronic complications of diabetes are macrovascular complications (cardiovascular disease, cerebrovascular disease, and peripheral vascular disease) and microvascular complications (retinopathy, nephropathy, and neuropathy).[5,7] The duration of diabetes and state of metabolic control contribute significantly to the development of long-term complications.[5,7] Diabetes is the independent risk factor for cardiovascular disease, including myocardial infarction and congestive heart failure; indeed, cardiovascular disease is the leading cause of mortality in patients with diabetes.[5,7,11,13] The microvascular complications of diabetes, though having a less mortality

Division of Endocrinology, Diabetes and Metabolism, University of Tennessee Health Science Center, Memphis, TN 38163, USA
* Corresponding author. Division of Endocrinology, Diabetes and Metabolism, University of Tennessee Health Science Center, 920 Madison Avenue, Memphis, TN 38163.
E-mail address: sdj@uthsc.edu

Orthop Clin N Am 54 (2023) 327–340
https://doi.org/10.1016/j.ocl.2023.02.005
0030-5898/23/

impact, do considerably affect morbidity and quality of life. According to the Centers for Disease Control and Prevention, diabetes is the predominant cause of new cases of blindness among adults aged 18 to 64 years.[1] Approximately 12% of people with diabetes aged 18 years or older reported advanced retinopathy or blindness in 2019.[1] Furthermore, diabetes is the leading cause of end-stage renal disease.[1,10] Approximately 40% of adults aged 18 years or older with diagnosed diabetes had chronic kidney disease between 2017 and 2020.[1] Of particular importance to the practice of orthopedic surgery, peripheral neuropathy affects 50% of adults with diabetes in their lifetime and is a major risk factor for foot ulceration and lower extremity amputations.[14,15]

Pathophysiology of Diabetes Complications

Several mechanisms have been proposed to explain the microvascular complications of diabetes, including genetic predisposition, formation of advanced glycated end products and other hyperglycemia-induced alterations, glomerular hyperfiltration, oxidative stress, and free radical generation, among others (Fig. 1).[7,16–18] One key property of organs targeted for damage is their inability to limit influx of intracellular glucose during chronic hyperglycemia. The resultant surge in intracellular glucose is linked to several mechanisms leading to end-organ damage.[17] In addition, impaired blood flow in the vasa nervorum and demyelination of nerves also contribute to the development of peripheral neuropathy.[18]

Unlike the direct link between hyperglycemia and microvascular complications, the mechanisms underlying macrovascular complications often are multiple, including hypertension, dyslipidemia, insulin resistance, hyperglycemia, cigarette smoking, sedentary lifestyle, and obesity.[7,12,18] Curiously, the presence of microvascular and macrovascular complications has been documented in some individuals with prediabetes, indicating the susceptibility of target organs to damage from exposure to sub-diabetic levels of glycemic burden.[19–21]

Diabetic Foot Ulcers

The prevalence of foot ulceration among people with diabetes in North America has been estimated at 13.0%.[15] The estimated lifetime prevalence of foot ulcers in people with diabetes is 25%, responsible for triggering approximately

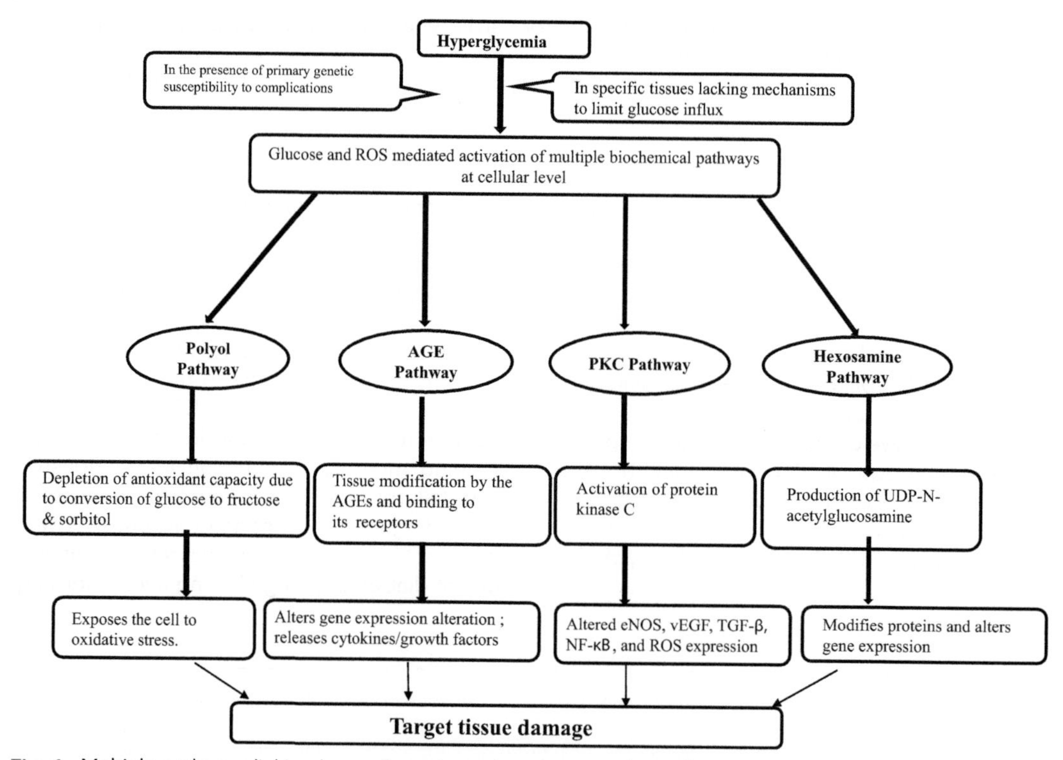

Fig. 1. Multiple pathways linking hyperglycemia to the microvascular and neuropathic complications of diabetes. AGE, advanced glycosylation-end products; eNOS, endothelial nitric oxide synthase; GF, growth factor; NF-κB, nuclear factor–κB; PKC, protein kinase C; ROS, reactive oxygen species; TGF-β, transforming growth factor–β; UDP, uridine diphosphate; VEGF, vascular endothelial growth factor.

80% of lower extremity amputations.[22,23] Moreover, foot ulcers contribute to approximately 50% of all diabetes-related hospitalizations and are associated with increased morbidity and mortality as well as huge economic impact.[24–26] Indeed, the estimated direct and indirect health care costs associated with diabetic foot ulcers and related complications exceed $1 billion annually in the United States.[25,26]

Numerous risk factors promote the development of diabetic foot ulcers (**Table 1**). Peripheral neuropathy and peripheral vascular disease, usually in concert with trauma, infection, and structural deformities, provide a pernicious milieu for the initiation of chronic ulceration.[14,22,23] Unfortunately, there is high rate of recurrence of diabetic foot ulcers; the recurrence rate has been estimated at 40% within 1 year after ulcer healing, 60% within 3 years, and 65% within 5 years.[23] Poor glycemic control is also associated with increased infection risks and impaired wound healing.[7,27] Hyperglycemia impairs wound healing by producing vascular super dioxide that inactivates nitric oxide, impairs angiogenesis, and causes vascular dysfunction.[28,29]

There is a compelling need to identify the risk factors for diabetic foot ulcers, implement active surveillance to recognize early lesions, and focus on preventive measures at distinct stages of ulcer development.

APPROACH TO MANAGEMENT OF DIABETES AND PREVENTION OF COMPLICATIONS

Patients with diabetes require a detailed history, physical examination, and comprehensive foot examination to identify patients at substantial risk for diabetic foot ulcers. Preventive measures should be taken early to avoid dreadful complications such as amputation.

Table 1
Risk factors for foot ulceration in people with diabetes

Diabetes-Related Risk Factors	Non-diabetes-Related Risk Factors
• Poor glycemic control	• History of prior ulcers
• Prolonged duration of diabetes	• Hypertension
• Retinopathy	• Foot deformities, trauma
• Nephropathy	• Older age • Poor foot hygiene • Smoking
• Peripheral neuropathy	• Peripheral vascular disease

NON-PHARMACOLOGIC MANAGEMENT

Lifestyle Interventions

The landmark study, Diabetes Prevention Program, showed a 58% reduction in the incidence of diabetes in the lifestyle intervention group compared with the placebo group regardless of the age, gender, racial, and ethnic subgroups with a minimum weight loss of 7% through moderate caloric restriction (500–700 fewer calories per day) and moderate intensity of physical activity of 150 minutes per week.[29,30] Similarly, the Finnish Diabetes Prevention Study showed a 58% reduction ($P < .001$) in diabetes incidence with lifestyle modification in the intervention group.[29,31] In addition, lifestyle intervention, compared with metformin or placebo, was beneficial in reducing blood pressure and stabilizing dyslipidemia, consequently improving cardiovascular risk factors.[32] Hence, lifestyle intervention is recommended during diagnosis as first-line therapy and adjunct therapies with anti-glycemic medication therapies if diabetes remains poorly controlled.[33] The elements of lifestyle adjustments include diabetes self-management education and support, medical nutrition therapy, physical activity, smoking cessation counseling, and psychosocial care.[34]

Patients with diabetes should be encouraged to engage in regular moderate intensity aerobic activity and resistance exercise for at least 150 min per week.[34,35] There may be a valid concern that people with diabetes who have developed peripheral neuropathy might have an increased risk of skin breakdown, ulceration, and infection with certain types of exercises. However, there is evidence that, with proper footwear, diabetes neuropathy did not lead to an increased risk of foot ulceration with weight-bearing activities.[36]

Along with physical activity, nutritional management constitutes a critical component of lifestyle intervention. The usual goal is a 5% to 10% weight loss in overweight or obese individuals, and a deficit of 500 to 750 kcal/d in caloric intake can result in the desired weight loss.[34,37]

The most efficient way to accomplish lifestyle intervention is through referral to registered nutritionists and dietitians along with direct counseling of patients by the clinician.[34] It is crucial to emphasize lifestyle interventions at every follow-up visit to reinforce the principles.

Cigarette smoking increases the risks for insulin resistance, peripheral vascular disease, ischemic limb, diabetic neuropathy, and cardiovascular morbidity and mortality of dyslipidemia and insulin resistance.[38–44] Smoking cessation is a cost-effective intervention strategy to decrease the risks of peripheral vascular disease, ischemic limb, diabetic foot ulcers, and amputation.[40] Clinicians should inquire about smoking habits and be aggressive in recommending smoking cessation interventions, including cognitive behavioral therapy, tapered nicotine replacement, and pharmacotherapy to decrease craving. Combining counseling with medications can be more effective than monotherapy alone for smoking cessation (Table 2).[34,40,42–46]

PHARMACOLOGIC MANAGEMENT

The treatment of diabetes includes oral and injectable agents. Historically, guidelines recommended the initiation of metformin after the lifestyle adjustments of diet and exercise. However, current guidelines recommend selection of the initial agent using a patient-centered approach, with consideration of comorbid conditions such as atherosclerotic cardiovascular disease, kidney disease, and heart failure (Table 3).[47] If hemoglobin A1c (A1c) control remains suboptimal, additional pharmacotherapies must be selected.[47]

As previously stated, metformin has been the mainstay treatment since the 1950s due to its efficacy (A1c reduction of 1%–2%) and weight neutrality. Although usually well tolerated, common side effects include gastrointestinal intolerance and possible vitamin B12 deficiency during prolonged treatment with metformin.[47,48] In the UK Prospective Diabetes Study (UKPDS), the subgroup of patients treated with metformin, compared with the conventional group, had significant risk reductions of 32% for any diabetes-related endpoint, 42% for diabetes-related death, and 36% for all-cause mortality.[49–51] Overall, the thiazolidinediones (such as pioglitazone and rosiglitazone) do not increase cardiovascular morbidity or mortality compared with standard glucose-lowering medications; in secondary analyses, pioglitazone treatment was associated with the reduced risk of composite all-cause mortality, nonfatal myocardial infarction, or stroke.[52,53] However, due to their adverse effects of fluid retention, exacerbation of heart failure, and reduced bone mineral density, thiazolidinediones should be prescribed cautiously.[53]

The dipeptidyl peptidase-4 inhibitors (such as sitagliptin, saxagliptin, and alogliptin) are well-tolerated oral agents with modest glycemic efficacy and generally neutral cardiovascular outcomes in randomized controlled trials. However, there might be slight within-class differences in the risk of treatment emergent heart failure, particularly in patients with high cardiovascular risk.[54] Sulfonylureas (including glyburide, glipizide, and glimepiride) have similar efficacy and accessibility as metformin. However, sulfonylureas are associated with a substantial risk of weight gain and hypoglycemia.[55] Although some observational studies have raised controversy about adverse cardiovascular outcomes with sulfonylureas, the UKPDS did not show increased cardiovascular morbidity or mortality with sulfonylureas.[55]

Two newer classes of antihyperglycemic agents have been shown to confer cardiorenal benefits in randomized controlled trials. The glucagon-like peptide-1 receptor agonist (GLP-1 RA) drug class (such as liraglutide, semaglutide, and dulaglutide) includes both oral and injectable formulations. Although generally well tolerated, these medications are started at low dosages that are slowly titrated up to reduce the risk of nausea, vomiting, diarrhea, and dehydration.[47] The GLP-1 RAs have been shown to reduce the risk of major adverse cardiac events in adults with T2DM with established cardiovascular disease or multiple risks factors for cardiovascular disease.[56–59] GLP-1 RAs are contraindicated in patients with a personal or family history of medullary thyroid cancer or multiple endocrine neoplasia.[56] More recently, an additional dual therapy consisting of a glucose-dependent insulinotropic peptide and a GLP-1 RA as a single (tirzepatide) was approved by the Federal Drug Administration, following demonstration of impressive A1c lowering effect of approximately 2% along with substantial weight loss.[60]

In addition to GLP-1RAs, the sodium–glucose co-transporter-2 (SGLT2) inhibitors (eg, empagliflozin, canagliflozin, dapagliflozin) decrease the risk of major adverse cardiovascular events, cardiovascular death, hospitalization for heart, and progression of chronic kidney disease in adults with T2DM with established cardiovascular disease or multiple cardiovascular disease risk factors.[61–63] The most common side effect is genital mycotic infection. Rarely, SGLT2 inhibitors can be associated with the increased risk of diabetic ketoacidosis, typically in the setting of insulin deficiency and decreased carbohydrate intake.[48,64–67] Owing to imbalance in amputation rates between active and placebo groups in an early trial, the US Food and Drug Administration issued a warning regarding the

Table 2
Available smoking cessation interventions

Therapy	Efficacy Versus Placebo	Methods	Duration	Cautions/Side-Effects	Contraindications
Behavioral intervention (cognitive behavioral therapy)	Increase quit rate by 40%–60%	In-person behavioral counseling sessions Telephone counseling Self-help materials	<20-min 1 visit and ≥20 min with >1 follow-up visit	Time limitation	
NRT (FDA-approved)	Increasing quit rate by 50%–70%	(Patch) 22 mg/day (Gum) 4 mg for 8–12 times/day (Lozenges) 9 lozenges/d for first 6 wk	Patch for 8 wk Gum for 12 wk Lozenges for 12 wk	Skin irritation Insomnia Vivid dreams Headache Mouth irritation Nausea Heart Burn	Contraindicated pregnancy
Bupropion (FDA-approved)	Increasing quit rate by >80%	150 mg twice a day	12 wk	Dry mouth Insomnia Headache Hypertension Increased suicidal risk in smokers aged <25 y	No human studies on bupropion use during pregnancy Liver damage Severe kidney disease Severe hypertension Avoid if seizure disorder or binge drinking
Varenicline (FDA-approved)	More than double the quit rate	1 mg twice a day	12 wk	Nausea Insomnia Headache Nightmares	Avoid in pregnancy

Abbreviations: FDA, Food and Drug Administration; NRT, nicotine replacement therapy.

Table 3
Commonly available antihyperglycemic therapies

Classes	Mechanism	Contraindications	Side Effects	HbA1c Reduction	CV Benefits ASCVD and HF	Renal Benefits
Metformin	Decreased hepatic gluconeogenesis	GFR <30	Nausea, diarrhea, B12 deficiency	1%–2%	ASCVD potential benefit	None
SUs	Increase insulin secretion	CKD	Weight gain, hypoglycemia	1%–2%	None	None
TZDs	Decreased insulin resistance	DKA, symptomatic CHF	Edema, weight gain, increased HF risk	0.75%–1.5%	ASCVD potential benefit	None
DPP-4i	Increase insulin, decrease glucagon	DKA	Hypersensitivity reaction, Potential HF risk with saxagliptin	0.5%–1%	None	None
SGLT2i	Increase renal excretion of glucose	T1DM, DKA, GFR <30%	Dehydration, hypotension, Euglycemic DKA in T1DM	0.5%–1%	ASCVD[b] HF[b]	a
GLP-1RA	Increase insulin secretion, decrease glucagon, slow gastric emptying	DKA Pancreatitis Medullary cancer	Pancreatitis reported though causality not yet established	0.5%–1%	ASCVD[b] HF None	a
Insulin	Binds to insulin receptor, inhibits glycogenolysis and gluconeogenesis	Hypersensitivity to insulin, during hypoglycemia	Hypoglycemia Weight gain	Variable	None	None

Abbreviations: ASCVD, atherosclerotic cardiovascular disease; CHF, congestive heart failure; CKD, chronic kidney disease; CV, cardiovascular; DKA, diabetic ketoacidosis; DPP-4i, dipeptidyl peptidase 4 inhibitors; GFR, glomerular filtration rate; GLP-1 RAs, glucagon-like peptide-1 receptor agonists; HF, heart failure; SGLT2is, sodium–glucose cotransporter-2 inhibitors; SUs, sulfonylureas; T1DM, type 1 diabetes; TZDs, thiazolidinediones.

[a] Strong evidence.

[b] Moderate evidence.

increased risk of lower extremity amputation with the SGLT2 inhibitor canagliflozin. This warning has since been retracted, following the accrual of additional data from follow-up clinical trials.[63,68,69] Systemic review and meta-analysis of published clinical trial reports did not show a signal of increased amputation risk with SGLT2 inhibitors.[70,71] In fact, emerging data suggest that patients with peripheral arterial disease experience higher absolute benefits from SGLT2 inhibitor treatment than those without peripheral arterial disease.[72]

Insulin is the mainstay of the treatment of type 1 diabetes (T1DM).[73] When orals or non-insulin injectables fail to optimize glycemic control in patients living with T2DM, insulin therapy must be initiated.

FOCUS ON LIMB PRESERVATION

Eighty percent of the amputations related to diabetic peripheral neuropathy are preventable with multidisciplinary care, reducing risks of amputation, hospitalization rate, and ulcer recurrence.[22] As already stated, diabetes accounts for more than 100,000 amputations annually in the United States, triggered by numerous risk factors including peripheral vascular disease, peripheral neuropathy, foot deformities, foot ulcers, trauma, and infection. With a better understanding of pathophysiology, advanced technologies, and the tools for optimizing glycemic control, there should be no tolerance for limb loss in people with diabetes.[7] Suboptimal care of early foot lesions increases the risk of amputation. The approach to limb preservation in diabetes practice can be segmented into primary, secondary, and tertiary intervention strategies (Box 1).

Primary Prevention

The successful prevention of the initial occurrence of amputation risk factors (peripheral neuropathy, peripheral vascular disease, infection) is desirable. The American Diabetes Association (ADA) recommends screening for diabetic peripheral neuropathy starting at the diagnosis of T2DM and 5 years after the diagnosis of T1DM.[74] ADA also recommends screening a low-risk patients with diabetes annually for neuropathy, peripheral arterial disease, and screening high-risk individuals with prior ulceration, amputation, and Charcot's joint more often at every visit.[74,75] During the foot examination, patients need a thorough foot skin inspection and neurologic evaluation, including 10-g monofilament testing, temperature, pinprick sensation, and vibration sensation using a 128-Hz tuning fork and palpation of pulses in the legs.[74] Patients should be educated about preventive foot care often.

ADA has emphasized achieving and maintaining an hemoglobin A1c (HbA1c) level of less than 7% for diabetes, based on the findings from the Diabetes Control and Complications Trial (DCCT) that showed intensive therapy to maintain HbA1c at 7% or less reduces diabetes-associated microvascular and neurologic complications by 34% to 76% compared with conventional therapy maintaining HbA1c at 9%.[7,75–77] The risk reduction for these complications of diabetes persisted and increased during the long-term observational follow-up study, the Epidemiology of Diabetes Interventions and Complications (EDIC).[78] The UKPDS showed similar long-term benefits from intensive therapy compared with conventional therapy in newly diagnosed T2DM, referred to as a "legacy effect."[79] Also, a 0.9% reduction in median HbA1c showed a 74% reduction in the risk of doubling serum creatinine level in UKPDS, which is beneficial in delaying the progression to end-stage renal disease.[7,80] In addition, the risks of development of any diabetes-related endpoint in the intensive treatment group were reduced by 24%, diabetes-related death by 32%, stroke by 44%, microvascular complications by 37%, and heart failure by 56% by controlling the blood pressure to 144/82 mm Hg compared with 154/87 mm Hg in the conventional group in UKPDS.[7,81]

Recent ADA guidelines recommend individualizing the blood pressure target based on cardiovascular risk, antihypertensive side effects, and patient preference.[11] Therefore, a blood pressure target of less than 130/80 mm Hg is the goal for patients with diabetes and hypertension at higher cardiovascular risk, whereas a blood pressure target of <140/90 mm Hg is the goal for diabetes and hypertension at lower risk of cardiovascular disease.[11] Angiotensin-converting enzyme inhibitors or angiotensin receptor blockers are the first-line therapy used for hypertension management in people with diabetes and coronary artery disease.[11] Similarly, the control of dyslipidemia must be optimized. Moderate-intensity statin therapy is recommended for patients with diabetes aged between 40 and 75 years without atherosclerotic cardiovascular disease, whereas high-intensity statin therapy is offered to those with cardiovascular disease or multiple risk factors.[11] Likewise, in the presence of atherosclerotic cardiovascular disease risk factors and diabetes, statin therapy can be considered for patients aged 20 to 39 years (Table 4).[11]

Box 1
Primary, secondary, and tertiary prevention for diabetic foot ulcers

Primary Prevention

- Take a careful history of symptoms of peripheral neuropathy and tailor the clinical effort toward documentation of the extent of any impairment.
- Optimization of glycemic control using the standard of care
- Screening at regular intervals for peripheral neuropathy using the 10-g monofilament, 128-Hz tuning fork, assessment of arterial pulses and more elaborate electrophysiological testing, as necessary.
- Smoking cessation assistance including counseling and medications
- Control comorbidities such as dyslipidemia and hypertension to reduce further microvascular and macrovascular complications
- Patients with diabetes must be educated to treat their feet with respect.
- Foot care includes
  - Advice to never walk barefoot
  - Encourage daily foot inspection
  - Emphasize wearing breathable loose footwear such as tennis shoes with non-constricting socks, avoiding tight-fitting silhouette shoes.
  - Avoid loose dressing
  - Avoid slippery floor
  - Avoid undertaking self-pedicure to prevent early lesions from infection and progressing into a pre-gangrenous foot ulcer

Secondary Prevention

- Prompt care by appropriate clinical staff is mandatory and much better than home remedies in the presence of skin breach, early abrasions, or superficial lesions in lower extremities.
- In the presence of bunion or other foot lesions, the patient with diabetes is best served by referral to the podiatrist for early management instead of trying home remedies.
- Use a broad-spectrum antibiotic coverage for infected foot lesions due to the polymicrobial nature of the infection in diabetic foot ulcers.
- Local management, including wound debridement, cast walkers for reducing the weight-bearing pressure on the affected foot, moist dressings for wound healing, and negative wound pressure therapy

Tertiary Prevention

- Revascularization of ischemic limbs can improve limb perfusion and consequently minimize the amputation rate.

In a recent study, the intensive glycemic control in T1DM early in their course was associated with significant risk reduction for all diabetic foot ulcers by 23% during long-term follow-up in the DCCT/EDIC study; however, the study did not confirm the risk reduction of amputation given few amputations seen secondary to the small power to detect associations.[82]

Secondary Prevention

The prevention of initial ulcer or recurrence of ulcer is essential in unfortunate circumstances where the risk factors for ulceration develop or in the presence of initial ulcer. Prompt care by appropriate clinical staff is mandatory and much better than home remedies in the presence of skin breaches, early abrasions, or superficial lesions in the lower extremities. Patients with neuropathy and risk factors for ulceration may benefit from well-fitted walking shoes or athletic shoes with adequate cushioning of their feet.[7,74] Custom therapeutic shoes are beneficial for patients with significant neuropathy, foot deformities, or previous amputation to prevent ulcers.[74,83,84] Infected diabetic foot lesions, especially with a history of prior treatment, antibiotic-resistant organisms, or severe infection, would benefit from broad-spectrum antibiotic coverage, given the polymicrobial nature of the infection in diabetic foot ulcers.[74,85] Management of foot

Table 4
Surveillance for long-term complications of diabetes

Diabetes Complications	Screening Techniques	Frequency	Target Goals
Cardiovascular disease(CVD)	Check blood pressure	Every clinic visit	Individualize target At low risk of CVD; BP < 140/90 mm Hg At high risk of CVD; BP < 130/80 mm Hg
Dyslipidemia	Check lipid profile	If not on lipid-lowering therapy, then at the time of diagnosis and every 5 y if <40 y or more frequently if indicated	Without known CVD: LDL <100 mg/dL With CVD: LDL <70 mg/dL, HDL >40 mg/dL in men, >50 mg/dL in women, TG < 150 mg/dL
Nephropathy	Spot urinary albumin to creatinine ratio GFR	Yearly Yearly	Albumin-creatinine ratio <30 mg/g in spot urine GFR >60 mL/min/ 1.72 m^2
Retinopathy	Dilated fundoscopy	T1DM: starting at 3–5 y of diagnosis; then yearly T2DM: at the diagnosis; then yearly	To prevent irreversible vision damage
Neuropathy	Feet inspection Comprehensive foot examination	Every visit Yearly	Intact skin Normal feet

Abbreviations: CVD, cardiovascular disease; GFR, glomerular filtration rate; HDL, high-density lipoprotein; LDL, low-density lipoprotein; T1DM, type 1 diabetes; T2DM, type 2 diabetes; TG, triglyceride.

ulcers is better provided by multidisciplinary teams, including podiatrists, orthopedic surgeons, infectious disease specialists, and wound care teams.[74,85] Diabetic foot ulcers may require debridement to remove the eschar and surrounding calluses to assist with wound healing.[83,85,86] Debridement can be achieved using different methods, such as sharp, chemical, and biological methods; however, due to insufficient data regarding the efficacy and the cost-effectiveness of different debridement techniques, more studies are required in the future.[86] Total contact casting for off-loading pressure from mid-foot and hindfoot ulcers has shown robust healing outcomes in treating diabetic foot ulcers.[85–88] Several dressings are available to aid moist wound healing and controlling exudation.[83,85] The adjunct therapy, hyperbaric oxygen, helps with wound healing by increasing angiogenesis and fibroblast proliferation and minimizing inflammation with oxygen flow; however, it has conflicting evidence regarding its long-term effectiveness.[85,86,89,90] Likewise, negative pressure wound therapy does not show consistent findings regarding potential benefits in diabetic foot ulcer.[85,86,91,92]

Tertiary Prevention

Patient with diabetes with a prior history of diabetic foot ulcer, prior abnormal vascular findings, peripheral vascular disease with prior intervention, and atherosclerotic cardiovascular disease would benefit from annual vascular examination (including ankle brachial index) and aggressive interventions to prevent toe, foot, below-knee, or any lower extremity amputation.[74,83,85] Patients with symptoms and signs suggestive of significant peripheral vascular disease should be referred to a diabetes-focused vascular surgeon for timely intervention and consideration of revascularization.[74,83,85] There has been conflicting evidence regarding the choice of revascularization with no distinct evidence favoring endovascular surgery compared with open bypass surgery.[83,93] Recent guidelines suggest that bypass surgery for patients with long-segment peripheral vascular disease may be preferable, though in most patients with diabetes and peripheral vascular disease, intervention choice depends on a range of factors, including availability of the vascular surgeon, extent of the arterial disease and infection.[83,94]

SUMMARY

The diabetes pandemic affects more than 537 million people worldwide and over 30 million adults in the United States. The risk factors for diabetes are vast and include hereditary and environmental contributors. The complications of diabetes can be prevented by optimization of glycemic control. The DCCT and other landmark clinical trials have proven that maintaining HbA1c levels of less than 7% can substantially decrease the risk of developing microvascular complications and the progression of preexisting complications.[76] Recent studies have shown that certain newer antidiabetic medication classes can provide cardiorenal benefits.[56–59,61–63,95,96]

The knowledge base of ortho surgery relative to diabetes includes clinical knowledge needed for managing diabetes. The key components are diet, exercise, and hygienic measures, including smoking cessation, promoting optimal health, appropriate use of antidiabetic medications, and goal setting to achieve and maintain target HbA1c. Also, HbA1c needs to be individualized to a particular patient risk factors profile, and a regular screening and surveillance for diabetes complications, including neuropathy, foot sensation, and peripheral vascular disease, should be done. Even in rare circumstances, where some of the difficulties have developed, there is an opportunity for secondary or even tertiary prevention, including arterial bypass surgery to revascularize the damaged tissues in lower extremity and prevent the loss of an entire limb.

Management of chronic morbidities includes dyslipidemia, hypertension, and enrollment in lifestyle management practice. Regarding physical activity, there is a clear correlation between aerobic fitness and longevity, which is mediated by myriad factors. Patients are encouraged to remain active even if they have lost their foot; it is rational to encourage these people to stay ambulatory and functional with a prosthetic limb to promote the longevity of the residual limb.

CLINICS CARE POINTS

- Patients should be monitored for diabetic peripheral neuropathy and other risk factors at regular intervals.
- Patients must be encouraged to work closely with their primary care physician or endocrinologist to optimize glycemic control, which is beneficial for preventing neuropathic complications.
- Lifestyle interventions, including diet, exercise, and smoking cessation, must be emphasized on every visit.
- Therapies with proven cardiovascular, renal, and heart failure outcomes are available and must be used appropriately to achieve glycemic targets.
- Emerging data showed higher absolute benefits from sodium–glucose co-transporter-2 inhibitors in peripheral vascular disease without increased risk of amputation.
- There are limited studies regarding the effects of antihyperglycemic agents on diabetic foot ulcers and their complications; therefore, future research is required to elucidate their role.

DISCLOSURE

D. Katwal has nothing to disclose. D. James has served as an investigator in clinical trial contracts with the University of Tennessee from Sanofi, AbbVie, Regeneron and Spruce Biosciences. S. Dagogo-Jack served as an investigator in clinical trial contracts with the University of Tennessee from AstraZeneca, Boehringer Ingelheim, and Novo Nordisk, Inc; has received consulting fees from AstraZeneca, Bayer, Boehringer Ingelheim, Janssen, Medtronic, Merck & Co Inc, and Sanofi; and has equity interests in Jana Care and Aerami Therapeutics.

ACKNOWLEDGMENTS

Dr Dagogo-Jack is supported, in part, by National Institute of Diabetes Digestive and Kidney Diseases grants R01DK128129 and R01 DK067269.

REFERENCES

1. Centers for Disease Control and Prevention. National diabetes statistics report. 2022. Available at. https://www.cdc.gov/diabetes/data/statistics-report/index.html. Accessed August 21, 2022.
2. IDF Diabetes Atlas 10th edition; International Diabetes Federation. Available at. https://diabetesatlas.org. Accessed August 22, 2022.
3. Davis J, Fischl AH, Beck J, et al. 2022 National standards for diabetes self-management education and support. Diabetes Care 2022;45(2):484–94, 95.
4. American Diabetes Association Professional Practice Committee. 2. Classification and diagnosis of

diabetes: standards of medical care in diabetes-2022. Diabetes Care 2022;45(Suppl 1):S17–38.
5. Nathan DM. Long-term complications of diabetes mellitus. N Engl J Med 1993;328(23):1676–85.
6. Virani SS, Alonso A, Aparicio HJ, et al. Heart disease and stroke statistics-2021 update: a report from the American Heart Association. Circulation 2021;143(8):e254–743.
7. Dagogo-Jack S. Preventing diabetes-related morbidity and mortality in the primary care setting. J Natl Med Assoc 2002;94(7):549–60.
8. American Diabetes Association Professional Practice Committee. Summary of revisions: standards of medical care in diabetes-2022. Diabetes Care 2022;45(Suppl 1):S4–7.
9. American Diabetes Association Professional Practice Committee, American Diabetes Association Professional Practice Committee, Draznin B, et al. 4. Comprehensive medical evaluation and assessment of comorbidities: standards of medical care in diabetes-2022. Diabetes Care 2022;45(Suppl 1):S46–59.
10. American Diabetes Association Professional Practice Committee, Draznin B, Aroda VR, et al. 11. Chronic kidney disease and risk management: standards of medical care in diabetes-2022. Diabetes Care 2022;45(Suppl 1):S175–84.
11. American Diabetes Association Professional Practice Committee. 10. Cardiovascular disease and risk management: standards of medical care in diabetes-2022. Diabetes Care 2022;45(Suppl 1):S144–74.
12. American Diabetes Association. Economic Costs of Diabetes in the U.S. in 2017. Diabetes Care 2018;41(5):917–28.
13. McAllister DA, Read SH, Kerssens J, et al. Incidence of hospitalization for heart failure and case- fatality among 3.25 Million people with and without diabetes mellitus. Circulation 2018;138(24):2774–86.
14. Ahmad J. The diabetic foot. Diabetes Metab Syndr 2016;10(1):48–60.
15. Zhang P, Lu J, Jing Y, et al. Global epidemiology of diabetic foot ulceration: a systematic review and meta-analysis. Ann Med 2017;49(2):106–16.
16. Greene DA, Lattimer SA, Sima AA. Sorbitol, phosphoinositides, and sodium-potassium-ATPase in the pathogenesis of diabetic complications. N Engl J Med 1987;316(10):599–606.
17. Brownlee M. The pathobiology of diabetic complications: a unifying mechanism. Diabetes 2005;54(6):1615–25.
18. Long AN, Dagogo-Jack S. Comorbidities of diabetes and hypertension: mechanisms and approach to target organ protection. J Clin Hypertens 2011;13(4):244–51.
19. Dagogo-Jack S. Primary prevention of cardiovascular disease in diabetic patients. Cardio Q 2006;12:20.
20. Brannick B, Wynn A, Dagogo-Jack S. Prediabetes as a toxic environment for the initiation of microvascular and macrovascular complications. Exp Biol Med (Maywood) 2016;241(12):1323–31.
21. Brannick B, Dagogo-Jack S. Prediabetes and cardiovascular disease: pathophysiology and interventionsfor prevention and risk reduction. Endocrinol Metab Clin North Am 2018;47(1):33–50.
22. Singh N, Armstrong DG, Lipsky BA. Preventing foot ulcers in patients with diabetes. JAMA 2005;293(2):217–28.
23. Armstrong DG, Boulton AJM, Bus SA. Diabetic foot ulcers and their recurrence. N Engl J Med 2017;376(24):2367–75.
24. Bandyk DF. The diabetic foot: Pathophysiology, evaluation, and treatment. Semin Vasc Surg 2018;31(2–4):43–8.
25. American Diabetes Association. Consensus Development Conference on Diabetic Foot Wound Care: 7-8 April 1999, Boston, Massachusetts. American Diabetes Association. Diabetes Care 1999;22(8):1354–60.
26. Wukich DK, Raspovic KM, Suder NC. Patients With Diabetic Foot Disease Fear Major Lower-Extremity Amputation More Than Death. Foot Ankle Spec 2018;11(1):17–21.
27. Selvin E, Lazo M, Chen Y, et al. Diabetes mellitus, prediabetes, and incidence of subclinical myocardial damage. Circulation 2014;130(16):1374–82.
28. Dagogo-Jack S, Egbuonu N, Edeoga C. Principles and practice of nonpharmacological interventions to reduce cardiometabolic risk. Med Princ Pract 2010;19(3):167–75.
29. Nyenwe EA, Dagogo-Jack S. Metabolic syndrome, prediabetes and the science of primary prevention. Minerva Endocrinol 2011;36(2):129–45.
30. Knowler WC, Barrett-Connor E, Fowler SE, et al. Reduction in the incidence of type 2 diabetes with lifestyle intervention or metformin. N Engl J Med 2002;346(6):393–403.
31. Tuomilehto J, Lindström J, Eriksson JG, et al. Prevention of type 2 diabetes mellitus by changes in lifestyle among subjects with impaired glucose tolerance. N Engl J Med 2001;344(18):1343–50.
32. Ratner R, Goldberg R, Haffner S, et al. Impact of intensive lifestyle and metformin therapy on cardiovascular disease risk factors in the diabetes prevention program. Diabetes Care 2005;28(4):888–94.
33. Davies MJ, D'Alessio DA, Fradkin J, et al. Management of hyperglycemia in type 2 diabetes, 2018. a consensus report by the American Diabetes Association (ADA) and the European Association for the Study of Diabetes (EASD). Diabetes Care 2018;41(12):2669–701.

34. American Diabetes Association. 4. Lifestyle management: standards of medical care in diabetes-2018. Diabetes Care 2018;41(Suppl 1):S38–50.
35. Colberg SR, Sigal RJ, Yardley JE, et al. Physical activity/ exercise and diabetes: a position statement of the American Diabetes Association. Diabetes Care 2016;39(11):2065–79.
36. Lemaster JW, Reiber GE, Smith DG, et al. Daily weight-bearing activity does not increase the risk of diabetic foot ulcers. Med Sci Sports Exerc 2003;35(7):1093–9.
37. Garvey WT, Mechanick JI, Brett EM, et al. American Association of Clinical Endocrinologists and American College of Endocrinology comprehensive clinical practice guidelines for medical care of patients with obesity. Endocr Pract 2016;22(Suppl 3):1–203.
38. Khaw KT, Wareham N, Bingham S, et al. Association of hemoglobin A1c with cardiovascular disease and mortality in adults: the European prospective investigation into cancer in Norfolk. Ann Intern Med 2004;141(6):413–20.
39. Kong C, Nimmo L, Elatrozy T, et al. Smoking is associated with increased hepatic lipase activity, insulin resistance, dyslipidaemia and early atherosclerosis in type 2 diabetes. Atherosclerosis 2001; 156(2):373–8.
40. Xia N, Morteza A, Yang F, et al. Review of the role of cigarette smoking in diabetic foot. J Diabetes Investig 2019;10(2):202–15.
41. Tesfaye S, Chaturvedi N, Eaton SE, et al. Vascular risk factors and diabetic neuropathy. N Engl J Med 2005;352(4):341–50.
42. Barua RS, Rigotti NA, Benowitz NL, et al. 2018 ACC expert consensus decision pathway on tobacco cessation treatment: a report of the American College of Cardiology task force on clinical expert consensus documents. J Am Coll Cardiol 2018; 72(25):3332–65.
43. Siu AL, Preventive Services Task Force US. Behavioral and pharmacotherapy interventions for tobacco smoking cessation in adults, including pregnant women: U.S. preventive services task force recommendation statement. Ann Intern Med 2015;163(8):622–34.
44. Rigotti NA. Strategies to help a smoker who is struggling to quit. JAMA 2012;308(15):1573–80.
45. Handelsman Y, Anderson JE, Bakris GL, et al. DCRM Multispecialty Practice Recommendations for the management of diabetes, cardiorenal, and metabolic diseases. J Diabetes Complications 2022;36(2):108101.
46. American Diabetes Association. 6. Glycemic targets: standards of medical care in diabetes-2021. Diabetes Care 2021;44(Suppl 1):S73–84.
47. American Diabetes Association Professional Practice Committee. 9. Pharmacologic approaches to glycemic treatment: Standards of Medical Care in Diabetes—2022. Diabetes Care 2022;45(Suppl. 1): S125–43.
48. Davies MJ, Aroda VR, Collins BS, et al. Management of hyperglycemia in type 2 diabetes, 2022. a consensus report by the American Diabetes Association (ADA) and the European Association for the Study of Diabetes (EASD). Diabetes Care 2022; 45(11):2753–86.
49. Inzucchi SE, Bergenstal RM, Buse JB, et al. Management of hyperglycemia in type 2 diabetes, 2015: a patient-centered approach: update to a position statement of the American Diabetes Association and the European Association for the Study of Diabetes. Diabetes Care 2015;38(1):140–9.
50. Effect of intensive blood-glucose control with metformin on complications in overweight patients with type 2 diabetes (UKPDS 34). UK Prospective Diabetes Study (UKPDS) Group. Lancet 1998; 352(9131):854–65.
51. Deacon CF, Lebovitz HE. Comparative review of dipeptidyl peptidase-4 inhibitors and sulphonylureas. Diabetes Obes Metab 2016;18(4):333–47.
52. Dormandy JA, Charbonnel B, Eckland DJ, et al. Secondary prevention of macrovascular events in patients with type 2 diabetes in the PROactive Study (PROspective pioglitAzone Clinical Trial In macroVascular Events): a randomised controlled trial. Lancet 2005;366(9493):1279–89.
53. Home PD, Pocock SJ, Beck-Nielsen H, et al. Rosiglitazone evaluated for cardiovascular outcomes in oral agent combination therapy for type 2 diabetes (RECORD): a multicentre, randomised, open-label trial. Lancet 2009;373(9681):2125–35.
54. Kongwatcharapong J, Dilokthornsakul P, Nathisuwan S, et al. Effect of dipeptidyl peptidase-4 inhibitors on heart failure: a meta-analysis of randomized clinical trials. Int J Cardiol 2016;211:88–95.
55. Abdelmoneim AS, Eurich DT, Light PE, et al. Cardiovascular safety of sulphonylureas: over 40 years of continuous controversy without an answer. Diabetes Obes Metab 2015;17(6):523–32.
56. Nauck MA, Quast DR, Wefers J, et al. GLP-1 receptor agonists in the treatment of type 2 diabetes - state-of-the-art. Mol Metab 2021;46:101102.
57. Marso SP, Bain SC, Consoli A, et al. Semaglutide and cardiovascular outcomes in patients with type 2 diabetes. N Engl J Med 2016;375(19):1834–44.
58. Marso SP, Daniels GH, Brown-Frandsen K, et al. Liraglutide and cardiovascular outcomes in type 2 diabetes. N Engl J Med 2016;375(4):311–22.
59. Crowley MJ, McGuire DK, Alexopoulos AS, et al. Effects of liraglutide on cardiovascular outcomes in type 2 diabetes patients with and without baseline metformin use: post hoc analyses of the LEADER trial. Diabetes Care 2020;43(9):e108–10.

60. Karagiannis T, Avgerinos I, Liakos A, et al. Management of type 2 diabetes with the dual GIP/GLP-1 receptor agonist tirzepatide: a systematic review and meta-analysis. Diabetologia 2022;65(8):1251–61.
61. Wanner C, Inzucchi SE, Lachin JM, et al. Empagliflozin and progression of kidney disease in type 2 diabetes. N Engl J Med 2016;375(4):323–34.
62. Zinman B, Wanner C, Lachin JM, et al. Empagliflozin, cardiovascular outcomes, and mortality in type 2 diabetes. N Engl J Med 2015;373(22):2117–28.
63. Neal B, Perkovic V, Mahaffey KW, et al. Canagliflozin and cardiovascular and renal events in type 2 diabetes. N Engl J Med 2017;377(7):644–57.
64. Peters AL, Buschur EO, Buse JB, et al. Euglycemic diabetic ketoacidosis: a potential complication of treatment with sodium-glucose cotransporter 2 inhibition. Diabetes Care 2015;38(9):1687–93.
65. Ingelheim Boehringer. Prescribing information for JARDIANCE. Ingelheim am Rhein, Germany. 2022. Available at. https://www.boehringeringelheim.us/sites/us/files/documents/jardiance.pdf. Accessed November 15, 2022.
66. Janssen. Prescribing information for INVOKANA. Beerse, Belgium, Janssen. 2020. Available at: https://www.janssenlabels.com/package-insert/product-monograph/prescribing-information/INVOKANA-pi.pdf. Accessed November 15, 2022.
67. AstraZeneca. Prescribing information for FARXIGA. Wilmington, DE, 2021. Available at: https://medical-information.astrazeneca-us.com/home/prescribing-information/farxiga-pi.html. Accessed November 15, 2022.
68. Chang HY, Singh S, Mansour O, et al. Association between sodium-glucose cotransporter 2 inhibitors and lower extremity amputation among patients with type 2 diabetes. JAMA Intern Med 2018;178(9):1190–8.
69. Janssen. Prescribing information for INVOKANA. Beerse, Belgium. Janssen; 2020. Available at: https://www.fda.gov/drugs/drug-safety-and-availability/fda-removes-boxed-warning-about-risk-leg-and-foot-amputations-diabetes-medicine-canagliflozin. Accessed November 15,2022.
70. Qian BB, Chen Q, Li L, et al. Association between combined treatment with SGLT2 inhibitors and metformin for type 2 diabetes mellitus on fracture risk: a meta-analysis of randomized controlled trials. Osteoporos Int 2020;31(12):2313–20.
71. Dorsey-Treviño EG, González-González JG, Alvarez-Villalobos N, et al. Sodium-glucose cotransporter 2 (SGLT-2) inhibitors and microvascular outcomes in patients with type 2 diabetes: systematic review and meta-analysis. J Endocrinol Invest 2020;43(3):289–304.
72. Barraclough JY, Yu J, Figtree GA, et al. Cardiovascular and renal outcomes with canagliflozin in patients with peripheral arterial disease: Data from the CANVAS Program and CREDENCE trial. Diabetes Obes Metab 2022;24(6):1072–83.
73. American Diabetes Association. 9. Pharmacologic approaches to glycemic treatment: standards of medical care in diabetes-2021. Diabetes Care 2021;44(Suppl 1):S111–24.
74. American Diabetes Association Professional Practice Committee, Draznin B, Aroda VR, et al. 12. Retinopathy, Neuropathy, and Foot care: standards of medical care in diabetes-2022. Diabetes Care 2022;45(Suppl 1):S185–94.
75. Bus SA, Lavery LA, Monteiro-Soares M, et al. Guidelines on the prevention of foot ulcers in persons with diabetes (IWGDF 2019 update). Diabetes Metab Res Rev 2020;36(Suppl 1):e3269.
76. Diabetes Control and Complications Trial Research Group, Nathan DM, Genuth S, et al. The effect of intensive treatment of diabetes on the development and progression of long-term complications in insulin-dependent diabetes mellitus. N Engl J Med 1993;329(14):977–86.
77. Nathan DM. Realising the long-term promise of insulin therapy: the DCCT/EDIC study. Diabetologia 2021;64(5):1049–58.
78. Lachin JM, Nathan DM, DCCT/EDIC Research Group. Understanding metabolic memory: the prolonged influence of glycemia during the Diabetes Control and Complications Trial (DCCT) on future risks of complications during the study of the Epidemiologyof Diabetes Interventions and Complications (EDIC). Diabetes Care 2021;44(10):2216–24.
79. Holman RR, Paul SK, Bethel MA, et al. 10-year follow-up of intensive glucose control in type 2 diabetes. N Engl J Med 2008;359(15):1577–89.
80. Intensive blood-glucose control with sulphonylureas or insulin compared with conventional treatment and risk of complications in patients with type 2 diabetes (UKPDS 33). UK Prospective Diabetes Study (UKPDS) Group. Lancet 1998;352(9131):837–53.
81. UK Prospective Diabetes Study Group. Tight blood pressure control and risk of macrovascular and microvascular complications in type 2 diabetes: UKPDS 38. UK Prospective Diabetes Study Group. BMJ 1998;317(7160):703–13.
82. Boyko EJ, Zelnick LR, Braffett BH, et al. Risk of foot ulcer and lower-extremity amputation among participants in the diabetes control and complications trial/epidemiology of diabetes interventions and complications study. Diabetes Care 2022;45(2):357–64.
83. Hingorani A, LaMuraglia GM, Henke P, et al. The management of diabetic foot: a clinical practice guideline by the Society for Vascular Surgery in collaboration with the American Podiatric Medical Association and the Society for Vascular Medicine. J Vasc Surg 2016;63(2 Suppl):3S–21S.

84. Bonner T, Foster M, Spears-Lanoix E. Type 2 diabetes-related foot care knowledge and foot self-care practice interventions in the United States: a systematic review of the literature. Diabet Foot Ankle 2016;7:29758.
85. Lipsky BA, Berendt AR, Cornia PB, et al. 2012 Infectious Diseases Society of America clinical practice guideline for the diagnosis and treatment of diabetic foot infections. Clin Infect Dis 2012;54(12):e132–73.
86. Cychosz CC, Phisitkul P, Belatti DA, et al. Preventive and therapeutic strategies for diabetic foot ulcers. Foot Ankle Int 2016;37(3):334–43.
87. Fife CE, Carter MJ, Walker D, et al. Diabetic foot ulcer off-loading: the gap between evidence and practice. Data from the US Wound Registry. Adv Skin Wound Care 2014;27(7):310–6.
88. Lavery LA, Higgins KR, La Fontaine J, et al. Randomised clinical trial to compare total contact casts, healing sandals and a shear-reducing removable boot to heal diabetic foot ulcers. Int Wound J 2015;12(6):710–5.
89. Stoekenbroek RM, Santema TB, Legemate DA, et al. Hyperbaric oxygen for the treatment of diabetic foot ulcers: a systematic review. Eur J Vasc Endovasc Surg 2014;47(6):647–55.
90. Ma L, Li P, Shi Z, et al. A prospective, randomized, controlled study of hyperbaric oxygen therapy: effects on healing and oxidative stress of ulcer tissue in patients with a diabetic foot ulcer. Ostomy Wound Manage 2013;59(3):18–24.
91. Dumville JC, Hinchliffe RJ, Cullum N, et al. Negative pressure wound therapy for treating foot wounds in people with diabetes mellitus. Cochrane Database Syst Rev 2013;10:CD010318.
92. Rhee SM, Valle MF, Wilson LM, et al. Negative pressure wound therapy technologies for chronic wound care in the home setting. Rockville (MD): Agency for Healthcare Research and Quality (US); 2014.
93. Hinchliffe RJ, Andros G, Apelqvist J, et al. A systematic review of the effectiveness of revascularization of the ulcerated foot in patients with diabetes and peripheral arterial disease. Diabetes Metab Res Rev 2012;28(Suppl 1):179–217.
94. Mills JL Sr, Conte MS, Armstrong DG, et al. The Society for Vascular Surgery Lower Extremity Threatened Limb Classification System: risk stratification based on wound, ischemia, and foot infection (WIfI). J Vasc Surg 2014;59(1):220–34. e342.
95. Wiviott SD, Raz I, Bonaca MP, et al. Dapagliflozin and cardiovascular outcomes in type 2 diabetes. N Engl J Med 2019;380(4):347–57.
96. Cannon CP, Pratley R, Dagogo-Jack S, et al. Cardiovascular outcomes with Ertugliflozin in type 2 diabetes. N Engl J Med 2020;383(15): 1425–35.

Preoperative and Perioperative Management of Diabetics Undergoing Elective Foot and Ankle Surgery

Patrick Cole McGregor, MD*, Ryan LeDuc, MD

KEYWORDS

- Diabetes mellitus • Orthopedic surgery • Preoperative optimization • Foot and ankle surgery
- Comorbidities

KEY POINTS

- Optimizing foot and ankle surgical outcomes in diabetics requires a multidisciplinary care team involving the patient, primary care providers, anesthesiologists, and orthopedic surgeons.
- Proper preoperative and postoperative glycemic control, regardless of the presence of diabetes diagnosis, is imperative to mitigate complications.
- Counseling of diabetic patients regarding their increased risk profile is an important part of shared decision making before elective surgery in this population.

INTRODUCTION

Diabetes is the most common metabolic disease in the world. The International Diabetes Foundation estimates that 1 in 10 humans worldwide will carry a diagnosis of diabetes by the year 2030 and 1 in 3 adults by 2050.[1] More than 20% of all surgical patients have diabetes as a comorbid condition.[2] Diabetes is a systemic condition characterized by abnormal carbohydrate metabolism. The vast majority (>90%) of cases of diabetes are classified as type II diabetes mellitus. In this disease process, the body undergoes physiologic changes resulting in a progressive loss of insulin secretion from the beta cells of the pancreas. Long-term complications of diabetes develop gradually with time and occur due to nonenzymatic glycation of proteins. End-organ damage is linked to cardiovascular disease, neuropathy, nephropathy, and retinopathy, among others.[2] Orthopedic surgeons are treating an increasing number of patients with diabetes and the associated complications owing to the disease process.[3–6] Orthopedic foot and ankle surgeons are tasked with several unique challenges in providing care to the diabetic population. Nonetheless, successful outcomes are still attainable when consideration is made for the unique characteristics of these patients. In this article, the authors discuss management strategies of diabetic patients undergoing elective foot and ankle surgery.

BACKGROUND

On a cellular level, type II diabetes mellitus is the manifestation of insulin resistance. Insulin resistance involves the dysregulation of the metabolism of energy substrates, primarily glucose. Insulin resistance occurs due to a constellation of factors, including inflammation, free radical formation, dysregulation of protein synthesis, hormonal changes, and mitochondrial dysfunction.[7] Insulin resistance renders cells unable to use glucose and leads to unused glucose to be deposited in the tissues, leading to end-organ findings of diabetes. These cellular changes lead to clinical manifestations

The authors have nothing to disclose.
Loyola Medical Center, 2160 South 1st Avenue, Maguire Center, Suite 1700, Maywood, IL 60153, USA
* Corresponding author.
E-mail address: mcgregorcole@gmail.com

Orthop Clin N Am 54 (2023) 341–348
https://doi.org/10.1016/j.ocl.2023.02.006
0030-5898/23/

of "metabolic syndrome," including hypertension, diabetes mellitus, dyslipidemia, and central obesity.

On a societal level, diabetes management is taxing on health systems. In 2017, more than \$327 billion were spent on diabetes management of the US population. One in 4 health care dollars spent in the United States is spent on patients with a confirmed diagnosis of diabetes, and of this dollar amount, more than half are spent directly on diabetic care. In addition, those diagnosed with diabetes have on average 2.3 times greater medical expenditures than nondiabetics. Aside from direct medical costs, there is an indirect financial cost of diabetes, with increased absenteeism in the workplace (estimated cost of \$3.3 billion), reduced productivity for those employed (\$26.9 billion) and those unemployed (\$2.3 billion), costly time away from work for disease-related disability (\$37.5 billion). Furthermore, per the most recent estimates in 2017, there are 277,000 premature deaths annually in the United States attributed to diabetes, which carries a societal economic cost of \$19.9 billion. This analysis also determined that the economic cost of diabetes increased by 26% over a 5-year time period, from 2012 to 2017, because of both an increased prevalence and an increase in per-person costs.[8]

PREOPERATIVE OPTIMIZATION

There has been a targeted effort from surgical specialties to optimize modifiable risk factors before surgery to minimize the risk of complications. Preoperative optimization programs have been shown to reduce length of stay, reduce postoperative emergency department visits, and increase rate of discharges to home postoperatively.[9] The American Academy of Orthopaedic Surgeons (AAOS) Risk Reduction Toolkit provides orthopedic surgeons with guidance on best practices for optimizing patients before elective orthopedic surgery.[10]

Determining the type of diabetes mellitus is imperative to proper management of these patients in the perioperative period. Type 1 diabetics require basal insulin at all times given their physiologic insulinopenia as a result of immune-mediated destruction of pancreatic B islet cells. Type 2 diabetics have a much larger spectrum of disease, and it is important to discern if they are an "insulin-dependent" diabetic requiring insulin or if they have managed their disease with lifestyle changes or oral medications only.

Preoperative glycemic control

Preoperative glycemic control is a common target for optimizing modifiable risk factors before elective surgery, with many institutions using hemoglobin A1c (HbA_{1c}) cutoffs to achieve before indication for surgery. HbA_{1c} is a marker of the patient's baseline glycemic control over the preceding 3 months. Much of the orthopedic literature comes from the adult reconstruction data on this topic. A recent meta-analysis reviewed 10 studies and concluded that there was an association with surgical site infection (SSI) and periprosthetic joint infection (PJI) in those patients with elevated HbA_{1c} levels.[11] The meta-analysis was limited by the fact that many of the studies used different HbA_{1c} percentage cutoffs (7.0, 7.5, or 8.0) and did not analyze HbA_{1c} as a continuous variable. Perioperative random fasting glucose has also been used as a marker for glycemic control in foot and ankle surgery. A perioperative random blood glucose level greater than or equal to 200 mg/dL has been associated with a statistically significant increase in the risk for SSI, among other perioperative morbidities.[4]

There is a wide range of HbA_{1c} "cutoffs" published in the literature that have been used as a way to determine patient readiness for elective surgery. Despite the abundance of literature, there is still no consensus on a cutoff that minimizes potential complications while still permitting diabetics to undergo elective surgery. Adult reconstruction literature from a study of patients in the Veterans Affairs system demonstrated that 15% of patients had their elective total joint arthroplasty postponed owing to elevated HbA_{1c}. Of these patients, 41% were unable to attain the goal HbA_{1c} within a period of time up to 3 years after cancellation.[12] Domek and colleagues[6] reviewed all elective foot and ankle surgeries in the Veterans Affairs system between 2008 and 2013 to determine the relationship between elevated HbA_{1c} and surgical complications. Their group found that the average HbA_{1c} for patients experiencing any complication was 6.29 compared with 6.11 for those who did not experience a complication ($P<.001$). Each 1.0% increase in HbA_{1c} portended a 5% increased odds of complications following elective foot and ankle surgery.

Nutritional optimization

Optimizing the nutrition of diabetic patients undergoing foot and ankle surgery is often overlooked in the lead up to an elective operation. Previous literature has shown that factors such as a lymphocyte count less than 1500 cells/mL, an albumin level less than 3.5 g/dL, a zinc level less than 5 mg/dL, and a transferrin level less than 200 mg/dL have been associated with increased risk infection and delayed wound healing.[13] The AAOS Risk Reduction Toolkit provides goal values for the aforementioned nutritional markers in addition to others to guide clinicians on when nutrition is at an optimal level for elective surgery.[10]

Preoperative cardiac evaluation

Cardiovascular disease is the ultimate cause of death in 80% of diabetic patients. Diabetes causes microvascular disease that affects the coronary arteries and places diabetics at higher risk of myocardial ischemia and cerebrovascular events.[14] The Revised Cardiac Risk Index (RCRI), a validated tool used to calculate risk of cardiac complications after noncardiac surgery, counts insulin-dependent diabetes as 1 of 6 major criteria that factor into the scoring system.[15] Other factors weighed into the RCRI include elevated-risk surgery (ie, intraperitoneal, intrathoracic, suprainguinal vascular), history of ischemic heart disease, history of congestive heart failure, history of cerebrovascular disease, and preoperative creatinine greater than 2 mg/dL. The RCRI has been validated in multiple studies, including a systematic review published in the *Annals of Internal Medicine*.[16]

Neurovascular evaluation

Preoperative vascular examination is paramount in diabetic patients undergoing foot and ankle surgery. All patients should undergo palpation of their pedal pulses, and if abnormal, should undergo further vascular studies. The presence of pedal pulses plus the absence of claudication symptoms has a 96% negative predictive value for large vessel disease. In patients without palpable pulses or weakly dopplerable pulses, noninvasive vascular studies are recommended, including following: ankle-brachial indices (ABIs) and toe pressures. ABIs can be unreliable in the diabetic population owing to calcification and noncompressibility of the vessels. Furthermore, ABI is a marker of macrovascular flow and does not measure tissue perfusion at the microvascular level, which can be compromised in many diabetics. Toe pressures are a more reliable test in patients with suspected microvascular disease.

An examination of sensation to the extremity is critical in the diabetic population as well. At the time of diagnosis of type II diabetes, 20% of patients are thought to be neuropathic, but this prevalence increases as time elapses and may be as high as 75% in diabetics.[17] The presence of peripheral neuropathy is a prognostic indicator for poor outcomes following foot and ankle surgery.[3,5]

Hospitalist comanagement programs

Increasingly, medically complex patients have led to an increase in the utilization of hospitalist comanagement optimization of many orthopedic patients. Early studies have questioned the improvement in quality of care and cost-effectiveness of hospitalist involvement.[18,19] However, these studies were limited by small cohorts and poor study designs. A 2009 article by Pinzur and colleagues[20] evaluating diabetics undergoing elective or semielective lower-extremity limb salvage or limb reconstruction procedures associated with diabetes demonstrated improvements in patient outcomes, including length of stay, associated hospital costs, and perioperative complications. The study demonstrated a model for a hospitalist comanagement system, which can be effective in reducing hospital length of stay despite a more medically complex patient population.

PERIOPERATIVE MANAGEMENT

Day of Surgery Medications

If the patient has an established endocrinologist or other primary care provider for their diabetes management, it is advisable to develop a plan for the medication regimen for the days leading up to surgery and the day of surgery. In many cases, it can be beneficial to schedule surgery for diabetic patients early in the day to prevent large fluctuations in blood glucose levels from remaining nil per os for prolonged periods.

There is a lack of literature on exact recommendations regarding day before and day of insulin management. However, many of the protocols involve reducing the dosage of both basal and bolus dosing of insulin to prevent hypoglycemia.

Perioperative Glucose Control

Regardless of diabetes status, perioperative and immediate postoperative glycemic control has been shown to reduce infection risk. The American Diabetes Association recommends a perioperative glucose target of 80 to 180 mg/dL. Previous studies have shown a reduction in mortality for those patients with more stringent glucose targets but higher rates of hypoglycemia.[21] Jämsen and colleagues[22] found that 25% of orthopedic patients in their cohort experienced severe hyperglycemia (defined as > 180 mg/dL) regardless of whether they had a diagnosis of diabetes. Expanding on this research, Mannion and colleagues[23] demonstrated that in nondiabetic patients experiencing hyperglycemia who were treated with insulin, the rates of a positive culture from any site and readmission were lower in comparison to nondiabetics with hyperglycemia who did not receive insulin. In addition, a series of 345 patients undergoing surgery of the foot or ankle found that those with a blood glucose level of 200 mg/dL or greater at any time in the perioperative period developed SSIs at a rate of 11.9%, compared with 5.2% for those whose blood glucose level remained less than 200 mg/dL (odds ratio [OR] = 2.45; $P = .03$).[4] Interestingly, in an arthroplasty database study, Chrastil and colleagues[24] found that HbA_{1c} level greater than 7.0 did not correlate with an increased hazard ratio (HR) of PJI, but perioperative hyperglycemia did correlate with an increased rate of PJI (HR, 1.44; $P = .008$). Numerous other studies in the total joint arthroplasty literature have shown that patients experiencing preoperative or perioperative hyperglycemia are at increased risk for VTE, stroke, urinary tract infections, postoperative ileus, hemorrhage, transfusion, wound infection, length of stay, and death, regardless of whether they carry a diagnosis of diabetes.[24,25]

The current body of literature, primarily from adult reconstruction, would suggest that regardless of the diagnosis of diabetes proper glycemic control is important to mitigate postoperative complications. Proper control of blood glucose appears to be as important, if not more important, than the presence of a diagnosis of diabetes mellitus.

Perioperative Hypertension

Diabetes and hypertension have been identified as risk factors for cardiovascular disease, and patients with both diabetes and hypertension have been shown to have a more increased risk of heart disease or stroke than patients with any of the 2 risk factors in isolation. Both hypotension and hypertension in the perioperative period have been shown to be economically burdensome for the health care system, as these lead to increased risk of stroke, kidney injury, and mortality.[26] Given the increased medical fragility of diabetic patients with hypertension and the propensity for adverse complications, careful consideration must be taken for hypertension management in diabetic patients in the perioperative period.

Practical Considerations

Although no formal guidelines exist, many practical considerations can be taken to optimize outcomes for diabetic patients on the day of surgery. First and foremost, DiNardo and colleagues[27] advocate for a multidisciplinary approach, with anesthesiologists being the most qualified and competent in managing day-of-surgery fluctuations in blood glucose level. This does require communication between the surgical and anesthesia teams in order to select the appropriate anesthetic that is optimal for the patient and for the surgery being performed. The use of regional anesthesia as opposed to general anesthesia should be considered when feasible and when regional methods prove adequate. In addition, consideration should be taken to schedule diabetic patients for the earliest cases in the day, as this will minimize the risk of hypoglycemic episodes. This also affords sufficient time for those in an ambulatory surgery setting to recover sufficiently and resume an adequate diet by mouth while still being monitored before being cleared for discharge home. Although merely suggestions, these are practical considerations that can be used by the orthopedic surgical team in providing care for diabetic patients.

POSTOPERATIVE CARE

Surgical Site Infection

SSIs are the largest contributor to the cost of hospital-associated infections. A meta-analysis of 522 studies investigated diabetes as a risk factor for SSI across all medical specialties. The OR for SSI in diabetics was found to be 1.53. Furthermore, the meta-analysis investigated preoperative, intraoperative, and postoperative hyperglycemia independent of diabetes diagnosis. The analysis found ORs for SSI to be 1.88 and 1.45 for preoperative and intraoperative hyperglycemia, respectively.[28]

In a 2017 article in *Foot and Ankle International* looking at the effect of the timing of preoperative antibiotic dose in clean, elective foot and ankle surgery, diabetes was *not* an independent risk factor for development of SSI, with rates of infection reported at 11.8% in diabetics and 10.2% in nondiabetics.[29] However, as the investigators point out, surrogate measures for disease severity were measured. Therefore, this article does not take into consideration the severity of disease status among diabetic patients, as it was only recorded as a binary value.

A meta-analysis by Shao and colleagues[30] reviewed the risk for SSIs after ankle fracture surgery. Their study involved 10 studies with 8103 cases. The overall infection rate in these cases was found to be 7.19%. The OR for diabetes-associated SSIs was 2.68 (95% confidence interval [CI], 1.39–5.16). The only higher risk factors in this analysis were open fracture (OR, 5.64; 95% CI, 1.92–16.56) and ASA Score equal to or greater than 3 (OR, 3.33; 95% CI, 1.85–5.98).

Wukich and colleagues[3] prospectively evaluated 2060 foot and ankle surgeries performed by a single surgeon and found that patients with diabetes and peripheral neuropathy were at 7.25 times higher risk to develop an SSI postoperatively compared with nondiabetic patients and 3.72 times higher than diabetics patients without neuropathy.

Because of the immunomodulating effects of diabetes, the immune system is unable to function well. This has been shown to result in an 80% higher risk of cellulitis, a fourfold greater risk of osteomyelitis, and a twofold increased risk of sepsis and death in diabetic patients when compared with nondiabetics with otherwise similar characteristics.[31] Furthermore, diabetics have a decreased ability to mount proper immune responses; diabetics are less likely to become febrile or develop a leukocytosis. Health care providers must remain vigilant to look for early signs of infection, particularly when treating diabetic patients. Oftentimes, one of the earliest infectious symptoms is worsening glycemic control.[32]

Althoff and colleagues[33] retrospectively reviewed almost 7000 total ankle arthroplasty patients and performed a logistic regression analysis to identify risk factors for postoperative infection and found that at 6 months risks factors for deep infection included the following: age greater than 65 years old, body mass index (BMI) less than 19, BMI greater than 30, tobacco use, diabetes mellitus, inflammatory arthritis, peripheral vascular disease, chronic kidney disease, chronic lung disease, and hypothyroidism.

Venous Thromboembolism Prophylaxis

There is good evidence to support that diabetic patients are placed at higher risk for developing venous thromboembolism (VTE). This is secondary to alterations in the coagulation cascade and fibrinolytic process, which leads to a propensity for microthrombi creation.[34,35] Following surgery on the foot and/or ankle, patients are often immobilized or given non-weight-bearing restrictions, which alone places patients at increased risk of developing a deep vein thrombosis owing to circulatory stasis, one of the 3 components of Virchow Triad. It has been demonstrated that diabetics with lower-extremity trauma are at a statistically significant higher risk of developing VTE (5.77% vs 4.60%; $P = .013$).[36] An analysis of diabetic patients included in the Worcester Venous Thromboembolism Study showed that diabetes was an independent risk factor for VTE. In addition, they determined that diabetics were more likely than nondiabetics to have a complicated course following VTE. Complications included long-term major bleeding complications and recurrence of VTE.[37] Wang and colleagues[38] discuss the importance of VTE prophylaxis in patients requiring diabetic foot care, as a history of VTE was found to be associated with increased all-cause mortality rates, a 1.6-fold increase in major adverse limb events, and a 1.4-fold increase in risk for amputation. Although limited evidence exists for optimal VTE prophylaxis regimens in diabetic patients undergoing foot and ankle surgery, the 2022 International Consensus Meeting on Venous Thromboembolism published in *Journal of Bone and Joint Surgery* gives a unanimous consensus strong recommendation for routine VTE prophylaxis for patients undergoing surgical debridement of diabetic foot ulcers.[39] Given the understanding of the underlying pathophysiologic changes and the implications of VTE, the importance of prophylaxis in the diabetic population must be recognized by orthopedic foot and ankle surgeons.

Resuming antihyperglycemic medications

For patients taking oral antihyperglycemic medications, instruction is given to hold their medications on the day of surgery, with the exception of metformin; patients are instructed to hold metformin beginning the evening before surgery given the risk of lactic acidosis. Postoperatively, guidelines have been set with regards to goals in random blood glucose levels. These goals include a target postoperative glycemic range between 140 and 180 mg/dL. When patients are admitted to the hospital postoperatively, the most effective way to ensure glucose control is via use of a basal/bolus insulin protocol. In fact, a randomized trial conducted in 2007 demonstrated this strategy to offer significantly better glycemic control than a sliding scale insulin alone.[40] The importance of maintaining tight glycemic control should be emphasized in the management of patients in the perioperative period and should involve the combined effort of the surgical team along with the anesthesia care team and the medical specialists. Hospital discharge is not recommended until the patient is tolerating adequate oral intake.[41] When this has been achieved, patients may safely resume their home oral antihyperglycemic regimen, although they should be instructed to closely monitor their blood glucose levels until levels have normalized.

Perioperative and postoperative antibiotics

Appropriate selection of antibiotic prophylaxis remains an important clinical decision to make in the care of patients in the perioperative period. Misuse of antibiotic agents is a contributing factor to the growing development of antibiotic-resistant organisms, which subsequently makes infection control much more difficult to obtain and increases resource expenditure. A systematic review of the literature on the use of prophylactic antibiotics in elective foot and ankle surgery demonstrated that, in the setting of clean, uncomplicated, and elective surgery for the foot and ankle, as well as elective surgery involving the bone and joints, antibiotic prophylaxis not routinely warranted, with "B" level of evidence.[42]

Postoperative antibiotics in the form of oral antibiotics to be taken at home after foot and ankle surgery have not been found to be protective against SSI. A study by Frederick and colleagues[43] retrospectively compared more than 3500 patients and found no difference in infection rates between patients receiving postoperative oral antibiotics for 3 days compared with those who did not after controlling for other factors. The investigators discourage the use of routine postoperative antibiotics in foot and ankle surgery.

Healing considerations

Given that diabetic patients are at a higher risk for wound-healing complications, the soft tissue envelope must be carefully inspected preoperatively and treated with great care intraoperatively. Skin changes common to diabetics that can impede wound healing include chronic venous stasis changes, swelling, and dry, inelastic skin. Preoperatively this can be addressed through aggressive edema management, often meaning delaying surgery until the soft tissue edema has decreased enough to safely make an incision. Postoperatively, vigilance is recommended.[44]

On a cellular level, hyperglycemia interrupts normal wound healing by impeding blood flow and tissue oxygenation, which can lead to endothelial dysfunction and a prolonged inflammatory state. In hyperglycemic states, neutrophils cannot phagocytose bacteria as efficiently.

As previously stated, optimizing nutritional status both preoperatively and postoperatively aids in the healing process. Malnourished patients have been shown to have a higher complication rate, including infection, hematoma formation, renal complications, and cardiac complications. Patients' nutritional status can be assessed preoperatively with routine laboratory values, including vitamin D, albumin, iron, and zinc. Knowing the status of these markers and optimizing them in the preoperative period is a critical step to minimize preventable complications.[45–47] One of the most common comorbidities of diabetes mellitus is obesity, owing to excessive and unbalanced nutritional intake.[48] Hospitalized patients with diabetes have 1.4 times higher rates of malnutrition than those without diabetes.[49] Another study assessing the rates of malnutrition in geriatric patients with diabetes showed a malnutrition rate of 21.2%, regardless of patient BMI.[50] The evidence supports the premise that preoperative nutritional status of the patient necessitates optimization in order to reduce the risk of complications, and this is even more pertinent in diabetic patients who have a higher propensity for being in a malnourished state.

Many of the procedures in foot and ankle surgery rely on bony healing to achieve the desired outcome. There is an established relationship between hyperglycemia and impaired bone healing in animal models. Diabetic fracture callus is relatively hypocellular and has lower rates of collagen synthesis in animals. These findings have been further corroborated in humans by small studies investigating nonunion and malunion risk factors in ankle fractures and elective arthrodesis of the foot and ankle.[6,51]

SUMMARY AND FUTURE DIRECTIONS

Caring for the diabetic patient undergoing foot and ankle surgery is complex. There are innumerable strategies to reduce morbidity for these patients; however, there is no single gold-standard protocol for preparing these patients for surgery. Because of the wide-ranging systemic manifestations of their disease, diabetic patients require more personalized care based on their disease state. Existing laboratory value cutoffs are imperfect and often overly stringent. Effective optimization involves a thorough medical evaluation to screen for potential comorbid conditions, which may alter patients' clinical course. Management of these comorbidities often involves consultation of other specialties as appropriate. During the hospital stay, hospitalist comanagement programs are effective tools for minimizing medical risk and should be initiated in the preoperative phase to allow proper evaluation of patients as well as to allow time for development of strategies for medical management of their conditions in the perioperative period. Future studies are needed to determine optimal antihyperglycemic medication regimens for maintaining tight control of blood glucose in the perioperative period.

Finally, thorough presurgical discussion with the patients and families is imperative. Ensuring that the patient understands that their diabetes imparts elevated risk for morbidity and mortality, regardless of optimization, is paramount to providing care in this population.

CLINICS CARE POINTS

- Maintaining perioperative and postoperative glucose below 200 mg/dL can reduce risk of post-operative infection in diabetic patients.
- Intact pedal pulses and absence of claudication has a 96% negative predictive value for large vessel vascular disease, however diabetics still may have microvascular disease that is occult on traditional vascular screening methods.
- Routine postoperative home oral antibiotics are not indicated following elective foot and ankle surgery, they do not provide protection against infection.

REFERENCES

1. "What Is Diabetes?" International Diabetes Federation - Home. Available at: https://idf.org/about-diabetes/what-is-diabetes/facts-figures.html.
2. Bodnar TW, Gianchandani R. Preprocedure and preoperative management of diabetes mellitus. Postgrad Med 2014;126(6):73–80.
3. Wukich DK, Lowery NJ, McMillen RL, et al. Postoperative infection rates in foot and ankle surgery: a comparison of patients with and without diabetes mellitus. J Bone Joint Surg Am 2010;92(2):287–95.
4. Sadoskas D, Suder NC, Wukich DK. Perioperative glycemic control and the effect on surgical site infections in diabetic patients undergoing foot and ankle surgery. Foot Ankle Spec 2016;9(1):24–30.
5. Wukich DK, Crim BE, Frykberg RG, et al. Neuropathy and poorly controlled diabetes increase the rate of surgical site infection after foot and ankle surgery. J Bone Joint Surg Am 2014;96(10):832–9.
6. Domek N, Dux K, Pinzur M, et al. Association between hemoglobin A1c and surgical morbidity in elective foot and ankle surgery. J Foot Ankle Surg 2016;55(5):939–43.
7. Yaribeygi H, Farrokhi FR, Butler AE, et al. Insulin resistance: Review of the underlying molecular mechanisms. J Cell Physiol 2019;234(6):8152–61.
8. American Diabetes Association. Economic costs of diabetes in the U.S. In 2017. Diabetes Care 2018;41(5):917–28.
9. Dlott CC, Moore A, Nelson C, et al. Preoperative risk factor optimization lowers hospital length of stay and postoperative emergency department visits in primary total hip and knee arthroplasty patients. J Arthroplasty 2020;35(6):1508–15.e2.
10. "AAOS Toolkits." American Academy of Orthopaedic Surgeons. Available at: https://www.aaos.org/quality/quality-programs/quality-toolkits/?embed_path=modexm%253DEmbedStart%2526toolkit%253DSurgical%252520Risk%252520Reduction%252520Toolkit.
11. Shohat N, Muhsen K, Gilat R, et al. Inadequate glycemic control is associated with increased surgical site infection in total joint arthroplasty: a systematic review and meta-analysis. J Arthroplasty 2018;33(7):2312–21.e3.
12. Giori Nicholas, PhD MD, Ellerbe Laura, et al. Many diabetic total joint arthroplasty candidates are unable to achieve a preoperative hemoglobin A1c goal of 7% or less. J Bone Joint Surg Am 2014;96(6):500–4.
13. Emara K, Hirose CB, Rogero R. What preoperative optimization should be implemented to reduce the risk of surgical site infection/periprosthetic joint infection (SSI/PJI) in patients undergoing total ankle arthroplasty (Taa)? Foot Ankle Int 2019;40(1_suppl):6S–8S.
14. American Heart Association. Cardiovascular disease & diabetes. 2015. Available at: http://www.heart.org/HEARTORG/Conditions/More/Diabetes/WhyDiabetesMatters/Cardiovascular-Disease-Diabetes_UCM_313865_Article. jsp/#.Wh_-eNKg_RY. Accessed 30 Nov 2017.
15. Lee TH, Marcantonio ER, Mangione CM, et al. Derivation and prospective validation of a simple index for prediction of cardiac risk of major noncardiac surgery. Circulation 1999;100:1043–9.
16. Ford MK, Beattie WS, Wijeysundera DN. Systematic review: prediction of perioperative cardiac complications and mortality by the revised cardiac risk index. Ann Intern Med 2010;152(1):26–35.
17. Guyer AJ. Foot and ankle surgery in the diabetic population. Orthop Clin North America 2018;49(3):381–7.
18. Auerbach AD, Wachter RM, Cheng HQ, et al. Comanagement of surgical patients between neurosurgeons and hospitalists. Arch Intern Med 2010;170(22):2004–10.
19. Huddleston JM, Long KH, Naessens JM, et al. Medical and surgical comanagement after elective hip and knee arthroplasty: a randomized, controlled trial. Ann Intern Med 2004;141(1):28–38.
20. Pinzur MS, Gurza E, Kristopaitis T, et al. Hospitalist-orthopedic co-management of high-risk patients undergoing lower extremity reconstruction surgery. Orthopedics 2009;32(7):495.
21. Leung V, Ragbir-Toolsie K. Perioperative management of patients with diabetes. Health Serv Insights 2017;10. 1178632917735075.

22. Jämsen E, Nevalainen PI, Eskelinen A, et al. Risk factors for perioperative hyperglycemia in primary hip and knee replacements. Acta Orthop 2015; 86(2):175–82.
23. Mannion JD, Rather A, Manifold S, et al. Postoperative hyperglycemia in patients with and without diabetes after major joint replacement: the impact of an enhanced glucose management program. JB JS Open Access 2021;6(3):e20.00172.
24. Chrastil J, Anderson M, Stevens V, et al. Is hemoglobin a1c or perioperative hyperglycemia predictive of periprosthetic joint. Infection or death following primary total joint arthroplasty?, J Arthroplasty 2015;30(7):1197–202.
25. Stryker LS. Modifying Risk Factors: Strategies that work diabetes mellitus. J Arthroplasty 2016;31(8): 1625–7.
26. Lizano-Díez I, Poteet S, Burniol-Garcia A, et al. The burden of perioperative hypertension/hypotension: A systematic review. PLoS One 2022;17(2):e0263737.
27. DiNardo M, Donihi AC, Forte P, et al. Standardized glycemic management and perioperative glycemic outcomes in patients with diabetes mellitus who undergo same-day surgery. Endocr Pract 2011;17(3):404–11.
28. Martin ET, Kaye KS, Knott C, et al. Diabetes and risk of surgical site infection: a systematic review and meta-analysis. Infect Control Hosp Epidemiol 2016;37(1):88–99.
29. Tantigate D, Jang E, Seetharaman M, et al. Timing of antibiotic prophylaxis for preventing surgical site infections in foot and ankle surgery. Foot Ankle Int 2017;38(3):283–8.
30. Shao J, Zhang H, Yin B, et al. Risk factors for surgical site infection following operative treatment of ankle fractures: a systematic review and meta-analysis. Int J Surg 2018;56:124–32.
31. Thomas R, Chou L. Diabetic foot disease. Orthopaedic knowledge update 5, foot and ankle. Rosemont (IL): American Academy of Orthopaedic Surgeons; 2014. p. 67–83.
32. Wukich DK, Hobizal KB, Brooks MM. Severity of diabetic foot infection and rate of limb salvage. Foot Ankle Int 2013;34:351–8.
33. Althoff A, Cancienne JM, Cooper MT, et al. Patient-related risk factors for periprosthetic ankle joint infection: an analysis of 6977 total ankle arthroplasties. J Foot Ankle Surg 2018;57(2):269–72.
34. Petrauskiene V, Falk M, Waernbaum I, et al. The risk of venous thromboembolism is markedly elevated in patients with diabetes. Diabetologia 2005 May; 48(5):1017–21.
35. Chung WS, Lin CL, Kao CH. Diabetes increases the risk of deep-vein thrombosis and pulmonary embolism. a population-based cohort study. Thromb Haemost 2015 Oct;114(4):812–8.
36. Chang W, Wang B, Li Q, et al. Study on the risk factors of preoperative Deep Vein Thrombosis (DVT) in patients with lower extremity fracture. Clin Appl Thromb Hemost 2021;27. 10760296211002900.
37. Piazza G, Goldhaber SZ, Kroll A, et al. Venous thromboembolism in patients with diabetes mellitus. Am J Med 2012;125(7):709–16.
38. Wang PC, Chen TH, Chung CM, et al. The effect of deep vein thrombosis on major adverse limb events in diabetic patients: a nationwide retrospective cohort study. Sci Rep 2021;11(1):8082.
39. Swiontkowski M, Parvizi J. International consensus meeting on Venous Thromboembolism. J Bone Joint Surg Am 2022;104(Suppl 1):1–3.
40. Umpierrez GE, Smiley D, Zisman A, et al. Randomized study of basal-bolus insulin therapy in the inpatient management of patients with type 2 diabetes (RABBIT 2 Trial). Diabetes Care 2007;30(9):2181–6.
41. Duncan AE. Hyperglycemia and perioperative glucose management. Curr Pharm Des 2012;18(38): 6195–203.
42. Modha MRK, Morriss-Roberts C, Smither M, et al. Antibiotic prophylaxis in foot and ankle surgery: a systematic review of the literature. J Foot Ankle Res 2018;11:61.
43. Frederick RM, Burnette H, Joyce M, et al. Efficacy of postoperative oral antibiotics in foot and ankle surgery. Foot Ankle Int 2022;43(9):1204–10.
44. Johnson JE, Klein SE, Brodsky JW, et al. Diabetes. Mann's surgery of the foot and ankle. Philadelphia: Elsevier Saunders; 2014. p. 1385–480.
45. Golladay GJ, Satpathy J, Jiranek WA. Patient optimization-strategies that work: malnutrition. J Arthroplasty 2016 Aug;31(8):1631–4.
46. Blevins K, Aalirezaie A, Shohat N, et al. Malnutrition and the development of periprosthetic joint infection in patients undergoing primary elective total joint arthroplasty. J Arthroplasty 2018;33(9):2971–5.
47. Deren ME, Huleatt J, Winkler MF, et al. Assessment and treatment of malnutrition in orthopaedic surgery. JBJS Rev 2014;2(9):e1.
48. Keskinler MV, Erbakan AN, Oguz A. MODY probability ratios in patients diagnosed with type 2 diabetes mellitus at a young age. Medeni Med J 2020;35(4):290–4.
49. White JV, Guenter P, Jensen G, et al. Consensus statement: Academy of Nutrition and Dietetics and American Society for Parenteral and Enteral Nutrition: characteristics recommended for the identification and documentation of adult malnutrition (undernutrition). JPEN J Parenter Enteral Nutr 2012;36:275–83.
50. Sanz París A, García JM, Gómez-Candela C, et al. Malnutrition prevalence in hospitalized elderly diabetic patients. Nutr Hosp 2013;28:592–9.
51. Beam HA, Parsons JR, Lin SS. The effects of blood glucose control upon fracture healing in the BB Wistar rat with diabetes mellitus. J Orthop Res 2002;20(6):1210–6.

Spine

Perioperative Management of Comorbidities in Spine Surgery

Zachary R. Diltz, MD[a,b], Eric J. West, MD[a,b],
Matthew R. Colatruglio, MD[a,b], Mateo J. Kirwan, MD[a,b],
Elliot N. Konrade, MD[a,b], Kirk M. Thompson, MD[a,b,*]

KEYWORDS

• Spine • Perioperative • Comorbidities • Complications • Management

KEY POINTS

- Medical disease burden is increasing in the United States in patients undergoing spine surgery.
- Poor management of medical comorbidities is associated with both major and minor complications in the postoperative period.
- Appropriate perioperative management of comorbidities is paramount to achieve optimal clinical outcomes.

INTRODUCTION

The number of spinal operations performed in the United States has significantly increased in recent years. Lumbar fusions have increased over 60%,[1] and cervical procedures have likewise shown a steady annual increase.[2] Along with these rising numbers, there has been a corresponding increase in the number of patient comorbidities.[3] As these trends are likely to continue into the future with an aging population, the need for appropriate and consistent perioperative management protocols will be paramount to optimize outcomes.

It has been well shown that an increasing comorbidity burden is associated with increased perioperative risk of adverse events and worse outcomes.[4,5] Although there is a lack of high-quality prospective data, the improved management of these comorbid disorders is expected to improve complication rates and postoperative outcomes. This review summarizes the literature and proposed the treatment strategies when applicable for common perioperative comorbidities in the United States.

OBESITY

Obesity rates continue to increase in the United States affecting an estimated 41% of the adult population, according to the Centers for Disease Control (CDC). An increase in spinal pathology, as well as associated clinical symptoms among obese patients, has been well demonstrated.[6,7] This occurs due to increased biomechanical loads translated through the spinal column, which can lead to infolding of the ligamentum flavum and increased disc bulging. Obesity is also a risk factor for epidural lipomatosis, in which excess adipose tissue in the spinal canal may lead to compression of neural elements.[8] Therefore, it is not surprising that a high number of patients undergoing spinal surgery are overweight or obese.[3]

Unfortunately, higher body mass index (BMI) has been demonstrated to be an independent risk factor for postoperative complications after spinal surgery. These include wound infection, deep venous thrombosis, cerebrospinal fluid leak, non-fusion, and mortality.[9–13] Patel and colleagues found a 14% major complication rate in patients undergoing spinal operations with a

[a] Department of Orthopedic Surgery, Campbell Clinic, University of Tennessee Health Science Center, 1211 Union Avenue, Memphis, TN 38104, USA; [b] Campbell Clinic Orthopedics, 1400 South Germantown Road, Germantown, TN 38138, USA
* Corresponding author. Campbell Clinic Orthopedics, 1400 South Germantown Road, Germantown, TN 38138.
E-mail address: kthompson@campbellclinic.com

Orthop Clin N Am 54 (2023) 349–358
https://doi.org/10.1016/j.ocl.2023.02.007
0030-5898/23/

BMI of 25, 20% rate with a BMI of 30, and 36% with a BMI of 40.[9] The increased risk of wound complications in obese patients has held true for not only posterior approaches but also with anterior approaches.[14]

There is a debate in the literature regarding whether clinical outcomes are negatively affected by obesity. Knutsson and colleagues found that a higher BMI was associated with higher dissatisfaction after surgery and inferior functional and quality of life outcomes.[15] Similarly, an as-treated subgroup analysis of the SPORT trial found less clinical improvement after operative treatment for lumbar disc herniation in obese patients with BMI greater than 30.[16] However, it should be noted that surgery still provided significant pain and quality of life improvement, albeit to a lesser degree. Interestingly, in further subgroup analysis of the SPORT trial, morbidly obese patients (BMI >35) actually experienced the greatest treatment effect for lumbar disc herniation and degenerative spondylolisthesis due to very poor outcomes with nonoperative management.[12] Conversely, other studies have demonstrated similar outcomes regardless of BMI in surgical treatment of adult degenerative scoliosis, anterior cervical discectomy and fusion, and degenerative lumbar conditions.[17–20]

Most previous work has included the significant proportions of patients undergoing traditional open procedures; however, recent studies have shown potential benefit to minimally invasive applications in obese patients. This is appealing as smaller incisions and minimal tissue dissection could lead to less wound-healing issues, a known complication in obese patients. Obese patients have been shown to have similar functional outcomes as measured by visual analog scale pain scores and Oswestry Disability Index (ODI), deformity correction, and reoperation rates after extreme lateral interbody fusion, and minimally invasive transforaminal lumbar interbody fusion (TLIF).[21,22] As minimally invasive techniques continue to grow, their benefit will need to be further studied in this cohort.

Surgeons must find an appropriate balance between operatively treating obese patients' legitimate pain and pathology against the increased risk in this group. Obese patients should be counseled directly regarding increased probability of reoperation, hardware failure, and potential inferior outcomes and encouraged to lose weight if possible. Strict BMI cutoffs have not been proposed, however, as the literature supports that obesity does not present a barrier to benefit from surgical intervention, and obese patients can derive long-term meaningful improvement.

AGE

There are an increasing number of both cervical and lumbar operations performed in elderly patients.[23] This is important because older patients have increased major and minor complications after surgery, and therefore, appropriate counseling and management are of utmost importance in these patients.[24,25]

Older surgical patients have been shown to have higher perioperative medical complications including delirium, urinary retention, venous thromboembolism, wound infections, and hematomas.[24,26,27] Structural issues have also been noted in those over age 65 with high rates of pedicle and compression fractures, hardware failure, adjacent level pathology, and development of proximal junctional kyphosis.[25] Age is also an important intraoperative consideration as it is one of the main risk factors for dural tears.[28,29] Using this knowledge to impact outcomes is difficult, though, as age is not a modifiable risk factor. Recently, literature has shown frailty assessment models to better predict outcomes of spine surgery than age alone.[30,31] These models take into account a combination of age and overall health to give a frailty score which can be correlated with complications and outcomes.

This knowledge can be used by surgeons to preoperatively plan instrumentation and technique as well as to provide realistic and data-driven expectations to this cohort of patients. Despite higher complication rates seen in both cervical and lumbar interventions for elderly patients, literature continues to show notable improvements in patient-reported outcomes and quality of life, suggesting that the benefits of surgery can often outweigh the increased risks for many patients.[26,32–34]

SUBSTANCE USE

Substance abuse can have a significant impact on both perioperative complications as well as short- and long-term outcomes after spinal surgery. Treatment with opioids has been shown in animal models to have detrimental effects on bone healing and can result in immunosuppression through reduced bacterial clearance.[35–37] Clinical studies have found opiate abuse patients to have significantly higher rates of spinal infections, pseudoarthrosis, 30 and 90-day readmissions, hospital length of stay, and need for revision surgery.[38,39] Duration of preoperative opioid use has been shown to be the most important predictor for continued use after surgery with chronic use greater than 6 months having the greatest risk for continued use.[40] However, even patients with non-sustained use for less than 90 days within 1 year of surgery were found to be at increased risk. Opiate-exposed patients are also more likely to require postoperative injections for pain control and have lower overall patient-reported outcome scores.[40–43]

Smoking tobacco also has many detrimental effects in the perioperative period. It is associated with higher rates of respiratory complications, wound infections, postoperative neck pain, delirium, and reoperation for adjacent segment disease after cervical spine surgery.[44–46] Current smoking is also associated with wound complications in lumbar surgery.[47] Fusion rates after both cervical and lumbar procedures are significantly decreased in smokers.[48,49] In addition, blood loss is higher in smokers than nonsmokers and is associated with longer hospital length of stays and higher costs.[50,51] Postoperative pain control is more difficult as tobacco smokers have been shown to require greater amounts of pain medication compared with nonsmokers.[52]

Cannabis use in the United States is rapidly increasing as it becomes legalized. Unfortunately, cannabis abuse perioperatively exhibits poor outcomes for spine surgery. It is associated with a significant increase in thromboembolic events, respiratory and neurologic complications, and sepsis.[53] In addition, cannabis abusers have greater difficulty with postoperative pain control and have been shown to require two times as many opiates as nonsmokers.[54]

Substance use must be carefully monitored and managed in the perioperative period. Every attempt should be made to minimize opioid use preoperatively. Likewise tobacco and cannabis smoking should be stopped before and for a minimum of 4 weeks following elective operations, particularly for fusion procedures.[49] All patients should have a health history screening preoperatively for tobacco and substance use with appropriate interventions started for cessation before proceeding with elective surgeries.

MOOD DISORDERS

The mind–body connection has long been thought to play a role in the development and severity of conditions of the spine and nervous systems. In the last 20 to 30 years, the literature has shed more light on psychosomatic conditions, bringing validation to many patients' struggles, and further reinforcing the importance of managing psychological disease concomitantly with surgical treatment. According to the National Alliance on Mental Illness, as many as one in five American adults will report symptoms of mental illness this year, with one in 20 reporting severe episodes requiring medical attention.

In a large, computer-modeled study addressing depressive phenotypes and their outcomes with spine surgery, it was found that depressive phenotypes had poorer reported quality of life, higher reoperation rates, decreased improvement from baseline, and more postoperative complications.[55] The study also found an inversely proportional correlation between severity of depressive phenotype and patient-reported outcomes. It has been reported that patients with self-described depression or anxiety have higher rates of lower back pain, disability, and lower quality of life in the immediate postoperative period. However, these results tend to become nonsignificant as more time elapses from the index operation.[56]

This highlights the need for preoperative risk factor identification and modification. Numerous studies have emphasized the importance of setting realistic expectations with patients preoperatively. One study demonstrated that adequate preoperative treatment of mood symptoms with both therapy and medication can lead to improved outcomes compared with untreated, matched cohorts.[57] Furthermore, it has been found that the degree to which patients can be optimized preoperatively is directly proportional to postoperative improvement.[58]

Office tools, such as the PHQ-9 and GAD-7, are frequently used in primary care offices to screen patients for symptoms of depression and anxiety. These tools are also useful in the surgical office as a gauge of patient mental state. Ultimately, mental illness plays a large role in our society and must be considered in the management of spine patients. The importance of honest and frank discussions with patients regarding mental health cannot be overstated. Similar to medical comorbidities, so too must mental illnesses be optimized and addressed before entering the operating room, as outcomes can be severely affected by untreated disease.

DIABETES MELLITUS

Nearly half of the US adult population is affected by diabetes mellitus (DM) or prediabetes, according to the CDC. DM can lead to increased medical and surgical complications in the management of patients across many specialties, spine surgery included. Physiologically, DM leads to delays in wound healing, reduced granulation tissue, and decreased macrophage function. These disrupt the inflammatory process which leads to biologic healing.[59] Numerous studies have shown that the diagnosis of DM carries higher reoperation, infection, nonunion, and transfusion rates, along with poorer outcomes and prolonged hospital stays in spine surgery.[59–61] The length of disease burden also correlates with poorer outcomes.[62]

Hemoglobin A1C level is an adjunct disease marker used to assess glycemic control over 2 to 3 months. Preoperative A1C $>$ 7 to 7.5% is associated with significantly increased risk of surgical site infection and deep infection requiring reoperation.[63] Therefore, screening is recommended preoperatively. The postoperative inpatient goals of care remain euglycemia and routine medication administration. In the immediate perioperative period, it is advised to hold home diabetic medications until the patient is consistently tolerating a regular diet by mouth. Sliding scale insulin should be used in the hospital setting to manage hypo and hyperglycemic events.[59] There has also been a recent trend to propose more minimally invasive surgery (MIS) strategies to mitigate the healing burden placed on diabetic patients, with a matched study showing superior outcomes in MIS TLIFs in diabetics.[64]

Even with elevated risk in uncontrolled diabetics, large studies have shown that diabetic patients show improvement after surgery as measured by ODI or Neck Disability Index and EuroQol-5D, albeit not at the same rate as matched nondiabetic patients.[65] When discussing surgical intervention, appropriate glycemic control should be achieved before elective procedures. Larger studies are needed to determine appropriate A1C cutoffs for elective spine surgery.

RHEUMATOID ARTHRITIS

Rheumatoid arthritis (RA) is a chronic, autoimmune disorder affecting joints throughout the body. The axial skeleton is the third most common site of involvement behind the hands and feet, and cervical spine disease affects 43% to 88% of RA patients.[66] Although spine involvement has been well reported, data are lacking regarding the use of disease modifying antrheumatologic drugs (DMARDs) in the perioperative period around elective spine surgery. However, the American College of Rheumatology and American Association of Hip and Knee Surgeons published guidelines in 2017 regarding the use of specific DMARDs and elective joint arthroplasty.[67] Methotrexate, sulfasalazine, and hydroxychloroquine can be safely continued throughout the perioperative period in a majority of patients. Consideration should be given to holding these drugs for 1 week preoperatively and 1 to 2 weeks postoperatively in elderly patients or those with medical comorbidities affecting drug metabolism. Leflunomide should be held for 1 to 2 days preoperatively and 1 to 2 weeks postoperatively. Cholestyramine can be used 1 to 2 days preoperatively to rapidly decrease blood levels of leflunomide's active metabolites. It is recommended to hold biologic agents for one dosing cycle before surgery and postoperatively until wound healing has occurred. Guidelines are shown in Table 1 for specific biologic medications.

Careful medication management is imperative in the perioperative period as continuation of certain DMARDs has been associated with increased risk of complications. Tumor necrosis factor-α (TNF-α) inhibitors have been shown to increase surgical site infections (SSIs) with a more recent retrospective study showing a 10x increased infection risk in patients taking a TNF-α inhibitor, irrespective of other DMARD use.[68] However, the risk of infection or delayed healing with continued use of rheumatoid medications has to be weighed with the risk of disease exacerbation, which can negatively impact rehabilitation and clinical outcomes, when planning for surgical intervention.

OSTEOPENIA/OSTEOPOROSIS

Osteoporosis is a quantitative, systemic disease characterized by decreased bone mass and skeletal frailty. Diagnosis can be made via clinical assessment after a fragility fracture, and measurement of bone mineral density (BMD).[69] The World Health Organization defines osteoporosis as a T-score of -2.5 or less in postmenopausal women and men 50 years and older and osteopenia between -1 and -2.5.[70] An expert consensus study recommended that patients over 65 year-old, regardless of risk factors, should undergo bone health testing using BMD before elective surgery.[71] They also concluded that younger patients should have their BMD tested based on certain risk factors as outlined in Box 1. It is recommended to get a dual energy x-ray absorptiometry (DEXA) before any fusion procedure in patients with RA and to start

Table 1
Perioperative medication management recommendations for biologic medications used to treat RA

Biologic Medication	Dosing Cycle	Schedule Surgery	Mechanism of Action
Abatacept (Orencia)	Monthly (IV) or weekly (SQ)	Week 5 or 2	CD80/86
Adalimumab (Humira)	Weekly or every 2 wk	Week 2 or 3	TNF-a
Anakinra (Kineret)	Daily	Day 2	IL-1
Belimumab (Benlysta)	4 wk	Week 5	BLyS (B-lymphocyte Stimulator)
Certolizumab (Cimzia)	2 or 4 wk	Week 3 or 5	TNF-a
Etanercept (Enbrel)	Weekly or twice weekly	Week 2	TNF-a, TNF-b
Golimumab (Simponi)	4 wk (SQ) or 8 wk (IV)	Week 5 or 9	TNF-a
Infliximab (Remicade)	4, 6, or 8 wk	Week 5, 7, or 9	TNF-a
Rituximab (Rituxan)	2 doses 2 wk apart every 4-6 months	Month 7	CD20
Secukinumab (Cosentyx)	4 wk	Week 5	IL-17
Tocilizumab (Actemra)	Weekly (SQ) or every 4 wk (IV)	Week 2 or 5	IL-6
Tofacitinib (Xeljanz)	Daily or twice daily	7 days after last dose	JAK (Janus Kinase)
Ustekinumab (Stelara)	12 wk	Week 13	IL-12, IL-23

The table lists the length of the dosing cycle, when to schedule surgery after the last medication dose, and mechanism of action for each drug. Recommendations are based on the 2017 ACR/AAHKS guidelines for elective joint replacement. AAHKS, American Association of Hip and Knee Surgeons.

osteoporotic patients on antiresorptive medications (bisphosphonates) or anabolic medications (teriparatide).[68] Multiple studies have found that untreated osteoporosis is a risk factor for hardware failure, screw loosening, reoperation and lower fusion rates, and appropriate treatment can decrease the risk of screw loosening and increase the fusion rates.[72–74]

It is recommended that a T-score below −2.5 is medically treated before spine reconstruction and that vitamin D levels be checked (<20 ng/mL associated with poor BMD) and appropriately treated. First-line treatments, after other causes of osteoporosis/osteopenia have been addressed, include teriparatide 20 mcg daily or abaloparatide 80 mcg daily. Second-line treatments are antiresorptive medications such as bisphosphonates or denosumab. Patient should be treated before elective surgery for a minimum of 2 months and treated postoperatively for 8 months with anabolic agents followed by antiresportives.[71]

HEART DISEASE

Cardiac comorbidities can lead to perioperative complications in spine surgery. However, there is a paucity of literature regarding the preoperative and perioperative management specifically in spine surgery. According to Guyot and colleagues, there is a 6.7% risk of perioperative cardiac complications in patients undergoing spine surgery, especially in the elderly and diabetic patient population.[75] Patients with a history of coronary artery disease undergoing a spinal surgery have an increased hospital length of stay, and increased risk of pneumonia, stroke, and death in comparison to control patients.[76] In patients with a diagnosis of congestive heart failure, there is an increased risk of pneumonia, stroke, and myocardial infarction when undergoing spine surgery.[76]

The American Association of Cardiologists defines elective spine surgery as intermediate risk and recommends that all patients undergoing elective spine surgery with a history of active cardiac disease should be evaluated by their cardiologist preoperatively.[77,78] In addition, the AAC recommends the continuation of all scheduled cardiac-related medications in the perioperative surgical period.[78] Prehabilitation in patients with cardiac disease, specifically congestive heart failure, can be considered as it decreases length of stay and increases satisfaction in patients undergoing spine surgery.[79]

Given the risk of perioperative complications in patients with a history of cardiac disease undergoing spine surgery, patients should ultimately

Box 1
Risk factors that should prompt bone mineral density (BMD) testing

Age 50–64

- Chronic glucocorticoid use (≥5 mg prednisone for ≥3 months)
- Previous low energy fracture of the hip or spine
- Metabolic bone disease
- ≥ Stage 3 chronic kidney disease
- High fracture risk calculated by FRAX (fracture risk assessment tool)
- Prior failed spine surgery (fracture, pseudarthrosis, instrumentation failure)
- Alcohol use (3 or more units per day)
- Vitamin D deficiency
- Current smoking
- Limited mobility, wheelchair based
- Current cancer treatment (known to impact bone health)
- Diabetes mellitus (>10 years and poor control)

Age <50

- Chronic glucocorticoid use
- Previous low energy fracture
- Metabolic bone disease
- Current cancer treatment
- ≥ Stage 3 chronic kidney disease

If any risk factor is present in a patient in the corresponding age group, a DEXA scan should be performed to evaluate bone health before elective spine surgery. If osteoporosis is identified, it should be treated before elective surgery.

be apprised of these risks during preoperative discussion of risk, benefits, and alternatives to spine surgery. Shared decision-making should be used when informed consent is obtained. Further research is certainly required regarding the management of cardiac comorbidities in patients undergoing spine surgery; however, patients with active cardiac disease should be evaluated by a cardiologist preoperatively, should continue cardiac medications perioperatively, and should be informed of risks specific to their conditions before undergoing any procedure.

KIDNEY DISEASE

There is limited literature regarding perioperative management of patients with renal disease undergoing spine surgery. However, patients with chronic kidney disease have increased perioperative and postoperative complications, including increased intensive care unit (ICU) admissions, urinary tract infections, postoperative delirium, and increased need for blood products.[80]

Friedman has published a comprehensive guide to the management of the surgical patient with renal disease.[81] It is recommended that patients treated with intermittent hemodialysis (three times weekly) undergoing elective surgery undergo hemodialysis within 24 hours of the elective procedure. In addition, preoperative laboratories specifically looking at potassium levels should be drawn within 12 hours of surgery.[81] Intravenous (IV) access is critical to any patient undergoing an elective procedure and can be difficult to obtain in a patient with chronic kidney disease (CKD). If peripheral IV access cannot be obtained and central access is needed, access should be preferentially drawn through the internal jugular vein as opposed to the subclavian vein to prevent stenosis.[82] In the preoperative period, attention should be paid to hemoglobin and hematocrit levels. In patients eligible for a renal transplant, transfusion of blood productions can lead to allosensitization, which can make future donor matching more difficult.[83] Consideration to an increased erythropoietin dose preoperatively may prevent need for intraoperative or postoperative blood transfusions.[83] Patients with kidney disease also have platelet dysfunction. Anticoagulation and antiplatelet therapy should be held in the perioperative period. Patients on warfarin or other anticoagulation should be considered for preoperative admission and initiation of heparin therapy, which can be held in the immediate preoperative period.[81] If bleeding is encountered intraoperatively, desmopressin (0.3 μg/kg), cryoprecipitate, and/or estrogen may be given to help control bleeding.[81,84] Patients with chronic kidney disease have delayed wound healing and consideration for staples kept in place for several weeks be considered over absorbable subcuticular sutures to allow for prolonged wound healing and decreased risk of wound breakdown.[85]

SUMMARY

As disease burden continues to increase in patients undergoing spine surgery, it is paramount to ensure appropriate perioperative management of medical comorbidities to decrease complications and optimize functional outcomes.

DISCLOSURES

The authors have no commercial or financial conflicts of interest or funding sources to report.

REFERENCES

1. Martin BI, Mirza SK, Spina N, et al. Trends in lumbar fusion procedure rates and associated hospital costs for degenerative spinal diseases in the United States, 2004 to 2015. Spine (Phila Pa 1976) 2019; 44(5):369–76.
2. Saifi C, Fein AW, Cazzulino A, et al. Trends in resource utilization and rate of cervical disc arthroplasty and anterior cervical discectomy and fusion throughout the United States from 2006 to 2013. Spine J 2018;18(6):1022–9.
3. Wilson LA, Fiasconaro M, Liu J, et al. Trends in comorbidities and complications among patients undergoing inpatient spine surgery. Spine (Phila Pa 1976) 2020;45(18):1299–308.
4. Worley N, Marascalchi B, Jalai CM, et al. Predictors of inpatient morbidity and mortality in adult spinal deformity surgery. Eur Spine J 2016;25(3):819–27.
5. Mannion AF, Fekete TF, Porchet F, et al. The influence of comorbidity on the risks and benefits of spine surgery for degenerative lumbar disorders. Eur Spine J 2014;23(Suppl 1):S66–71.
6. Teraguchi M, Yoshimura N, Hashizume H, et al. Prevalence and distribution of intervertebral disc degeneration over the entire spine in a population-based cohort: the Wakayama Spine Study. Osteoarthritis Cartil 2014;22(1):104–10.
7. Fanuele JC, Abdu WA, Hanscom B, et al. Association between obesity and functional status in patients with spine disease. Spine (Phila Pa 1976) 2002;27(3):306–12.
8. Theyskens NC, Paulino Pereira NR, Janssen SJ, et al. The prevalence of spinal epidural lipomatosis on magnetic resonance imaging. Spine J 2017;17(7):969–76.
9. Patel N, Bagan B, Vadera S, et al. Obesity and spine surgery: relation to perioperative complications. J Neurosurg Spine 2007;6(4):291–7.
10. Khalooeifard R, Oraee-Yazdani S, Vahdat Shariatpanahi Z. Obesity and posterior spine fusion surgery: a prospective observational study. Int J Orthop Trauma Nurs 2022;45:100920.
11. Kalanithi PA, Arrigo R, Boakye M. Morbid obesity increases cost and complication rates in spinal arthrodesis. Spine (Phila Pa 1976) 2012;37(11):982–8.
12. McGuire KJ, Khaleel MA, Rihn JA, et al. The effect of high obesity on outcomes of treatment for lumbar spinal conditions: subgroup analysis of the spine patient outcomes research trial. Spine (Phila Pa 1976) 2014;39(23):1975–80.
13. Varshneya K, Wadhwa H, Stienen MN, et al. Obesity in patients undergoing lumbar degenerative surgery-a retrospective cohort study of postoperative outcomes. Spine (Phila Pa 1976) 2021;46(17):1191–6.
14. Miller EM, McAllister BD. Increased risk of postoperative wound complications among obesity classes II & III after ALIF in 10-year ACS-NSQIP analysis of 10,934 cases. Spine J 2022;22(4):587–94.
15. Knutsson B, Michaelsson K, Sanden B. Obesity is associated with inferior results after surgery for lumbar spinal stenosis: a study of 2633 patients from the Swedish spine register. Spine (Phila Pa 1976) 2013;38(5):435–41.
16. Rihn JA, Kurd M, Hilibrand AS, et al. The influence of obesity on the outcome of treatment of lumbar disc herniation: analysis of the Spine Patient Outcomes Research Trial (SPORT). J Bone Joint Surg Am 2013;95(1):1–8.
17. Sielatycki JA, Chotai S, Stonko D, et al. Is obesity associated with worse patient-reported outcomes following lumbar surgery for degenerative conditions? Eur Spine J 2016;25(5):1627–33.
18. Sielatycki JA, Chotai S, Kay H, et al. Does obesity correlate with worse patient-reported outcomes following elective anterior cervical discectomy and fusion? Neurosurg 2016;79(1):69–74.
19. Brennan PM, Loan JJM, Watson N, et al. Pre-operative obesity does not predict poorer symptom control and quality of life after lumbar disc surgery. Br J Neurosurg 2017;31(6):682–7.
20. Truong VT, Sunna T, Al-Shakfa F, et al. Impact of obesity on complications and surgical outcomes of adult degenerative scoliosis with long-segment spinal fusion. Neurochirurgie 2022;68(3):289–92.
21. Changoor S, Dunn C, Coban D, et al. Does obesity affect long-term outcomes of extreme lateral interbody fusion with posterior stabilization? Spine J 2021;21(8):1318–24.
22. Coban D, Changoor S, Saela S, et al. Obesity does not adversely affect long-term outcomes of minimally invasive transforaminal lumbar interbody fusion: a matched cohort analysis. Orthopedics 2022;45(4):203–8.
23. Zileli M, Dursun E. How to improve outcomes of spine surgery in geriatric patients. World Neurosurg 2020;140:519–26.
24. Jalai CM, Worley N, Marascalchi BJ, et al. The impact of advanced age on peri-operative outcomes in the surgical treatment of cervical spondylotic myelopathy: a Nationwide study between 2001 and 2010. Spine (Phila Pa 1976) 2016;41(3):E139–47.
25. DeWald CJ, Stanley T. Instrumentation-related complications of multilevel fusions for adult spinal deformity patients over age 65: surgical considerations and treatment options in patients with poor bone quality. Spine (Phila Pa 1976) 2006;31(19 Suppl):S144–51.
26. Verla T, Adogwa O, Toche U, et al. Impact of Increasing Age on Outcomes of Spinal Fusion in

Adult Idiopathic Scoliosis. World Neurosurg 2016; 87:591–7.
27. Cloyd JM, Acosta FL Jr, Cloyd C, et al. Effects of age on perioperative complications of extensive multilevel thoracolumbar spinal fusion surgery. J Neurosurg Spine 2010;12(4):402–8.
28. Baker GA, Cizik AM, Bransford RJ, et al. Risk factors for unintended durotomy during spine surgery: a multivariate analysis. Spine J 2012;12(2):121–6.
29. Smorgick Y, Baker KC, Herkowitz H, et al. Predisposing factors for dural tear in patients undergoing lumbar spine surgery. J Neurosurg Spine 2015; 22(5):483–6.
30. Wilson JRF, Badhiwala JH, Moghaddamjou A, et al. Frailty Is a Better Predictor than Age of Mortality and Perioperative Complications after Surgery for Degenerative Cervical Myelopathy: An Analysis of 41,369 Patients from the NSQIP Database 2010-2018. J Clin Med 2020;(11):9. https://doi.org/10.3390/jcm9113491.
31. Mohamed B, Ramachandran R, Rabai F, et al. Frailty Assessment and Prehabilitation Before Complex Spine Surgery in Patients With Degenerative Spine Disease: A Narrative Review. J Neurosurg Anesthesiol 2021.
32. Youssef JA, Heiner AD, Montgomery JR, et al. Outcomes of posterior cervical fusion and decompression: a systematic review and meta-analysis. Spine J 2019;19(10):1714–29.
33. McCarthy MH, Weiner JA, Patel AA. Strategies to achieve spinal fusion in multilevel anterior cervical spine surgery: an overview. HSS J 2020;16(2): 155–61.
34. Glassman SD, Hamill CL, Bridwell KH, et al. The impact of perioperative complications on clinical outcome in adult deformity surgery. Spine (Phila Pa 1976) 2007;32(24):2764–70.
35. Chrastil J, Sampson C, Jones KB, et al. Evaluating the affect and reversibility of opioid-induced androgen deficiency in an orthopaedic animal fracture model. Clin Orthop Relat Res 2014;472(6): 1964–71.
36. Banerjee A, Strazza M, Wigdahl B, et al. Role of mu-opioids as cofactors in human immunodeficiency virus type 1 disease progression and neuropathogenesis. J Neurovirol 2011;17(4):291–302.
37. Ninkovic J, Roy S. Morphine decreases bacterial phagocytosis by inhibiting actin polymerization through cAMP-, Rac-1-, and p38 MAPK-dependent mechanisms. Am J Pathol 2012;180(3):1068–79.
38. Vakharia RM, Donnally CJ 3rd, Rush AJ 3rd, et al. Comparison of implant survivability in primary 1- to 2-level lumbar fusion amongst opioid abusers and non-opioid abusers. J Spine Surg 2018;4(3): 568–74.
39. Lui B, Weinberg R, Milewski AR, et al. Impact of preoperative opioid use disorder on outcomes following lumbar-spine surgery. Clin Neurol Neurosurg 2021;208:106865.
40. Schoenfeld AJ, Belmont PJ Jr, Blucher JA, et al. Sustained preoperative opioid use is a predictor of continued use following spine surgery. J Bone Joint Surg Am 2018;100(11):914–21.
41. Kalakoti P, Hendrickson NR, Bedard NA, et al. Opioid utilization following lumbar arthrodesis: trends and factors associated with long-term use. Spine (Phila Pa 1976) 2018;43(17):1208–16.
42. Kalakoti P, Volkmar AJ, Bedard NA, et al. Preoperative chronic opioid therapy negatively impacts long-term outcomes following cervical fusion surgery. Spine (Phila Pa 1976) 2019;44(18):1279–86.
43. Cook DJ, Kaskovich S, Pirkle S, et al. Benchmarks of duration and magnitude of opioid consumption after common spinal procedures: a database analysis of 47,823 patients. Spine (Phila Pa 1976) 2019; 44(23):1668–75.
44. Nagoshi N, Kono H, Tsuji O, et al. Impact of tobacco smoking on outcomes after posterior decompression surgery in patients with Cervical Spondylotic Myelopathy: a retrospective multicenter study. Clin Spine Surg 2020;33(10):E493–8.
45. Zheng LM, Zhang ZW, Wang W, et al. Relationship between smoking and postoperative complications of cervical spine surgery: a systematic review and meta-analysis. Sci Rep 2022;12(1):9172.
46. Lee JC, Lee SH, Peters C, et al. Adjacent segment pathology requiring reoperation after anterior cervical arthrodesis: the influence of smoking, sex, and number of operated levels. Spine (Phila Pa 1976) 2015;40(10):E571–7.
47. Martin CT, Gao Y, Duchman KR, et al. The impact of current smoking and smoking cessation on short-term morbidity risk after lumbar spine surgery. Spine (Phila Pa 1976) 2016;41(7):577–84.
48. Phan K, Fadhil M, Chang N, et al. Effect of smoking status on successful arthrodesis, clinical outcome, and complications after Anterior Lumbar Interbody Fusion (ALIF). World Neurosurg 2018;110:e998–1003.
49. Berman D, Oren JH, Bendo J, et al. The effect of smoking on spinal fusion. Int J Spine Surg 2017; 11:29. https://doi.org/10.14444/4029.
50. Wilson JRF, Jiang F, Badhiwala JH, et al. The effect of tobacco smoking on adverse events following adult complex deformity surgery: analysis of 270 patients from the prospective, multicenter scoli-RISK-1 study. Spine (Phila Pa 1976) 2020;45(1):32–7.
51. McCunniff PT, Young ES, Ahmadinia K, et al. Smoking is associated with increased blood loss and transfusion use after lumbar spinal surgery. Clin Orthop Relat Res 2016;474(4):1019–25.
52. Christian ZK, Youssef CA, Aoun SG, et al. Smoking has a dose-dependent effect on the incidence of preoperative opioid consumption in female

geriatric patients with spine disease. J Clin Neurosci 2020;81:173–7.
53. Chiu RG, Patel S, Siddiqui N, et al. Cannabis abuse and perioperative complications following inpatient spine surgery in the United States. Spine (Phila Pa 1976) 2021;46(11):734–43.
54. Goel A, McGuinness B, Jivraj NK, et al. Cannabis use disorder and perioperative outcomes in major elective surgeries: a retrospective cohort analysis. Anesthesiology 2020;132(4):625–35.
55. Boakye M, Sharma M, Adams S, et al. Patterns and impact of electronic health records-defined depression phenotypes in spine surgery. Neurosurgery 2021;89(1):E19–32.
56. Kashlan O, Swong K, Alvi MA, et al. Patients with a depressive and/or anxiety disorder can achieve optimum Long term outcomes after surgery for grade 1 spondylolisthesis: Analysis from the quality outcomes database (QOD). Clin Neurol Neurosurg 2020;197:106098.
57. Adogwa O, Elsamadicy AA, Cheng J, et al. Pretreatment of anxiety before cervical spine surgery improves clinical outcomes: a prospective, single- institution experience. World Neurosurg 2016;88:625–30.
58. Falavigna A, Righesso O, Teles AR, et al. Responsiveness of depression and its influence on surgical outcomes of lumbar degenerative diseases. Eur J Orthop Surg Traumatol 2015;25(Suppl 1):S35–41.
59. Michel M, Lucke-Wold B. Diabetes management in spinal surgery. J Clin Images Med Case Rep 2022;3(6).
60. Browne JA, Cook C, Pietrobon R, et al. Diabetes and early postoperative outcomes following lumbar fusion. Spine (Phila Pa 1976) 2007;32(20):2214–9.
61. Mobbs RJ, Newcombe RL, Chandran KN. Lumbar discectomy and the diabetic patient: incidence and outcome. J Clin Neurosci 2001;8(1):10–3.
62. Takahashi S, Suzuki A, Toyoda H, et al. Characteristics of diabetes associated with poor improvements in clinical outcomes after lumbar spine surgery. Spine (Phila Pa 1976) 2013;38(6):516–22.
63. Hwang JU, Son DW, Kang KT, et al. Importance of hemoglobin A1c levels for the detection of post-surgical infection following single-level lumbar posterior fusion in patients with diabetes. Korean J Neurotrauma 2019;15(2):150–8.
64. Narain AS, Haws BE, Jenkins NW, et al. Diabetes does not increase complications, length of stay, or hospital costs after minimally invasive transforaminal lumbar interbody fusion. Clin Spine Surg 2020;33(7):E307–11.
65. Armaghani SJ, Archer KR, Rolfe R, et al. Diabetes is related to worse patient-reported outcomes at two years following spine surgery. J Bone Joint Surg Am 2016;98(1):15–22.
66. Kawaguchi Y, Matsuno H, Kanamori M, et al. Radiologic findings of the lumbar spine in patients with rheumatoid arthritis, and a review of pathologic mechanisms. J Spinal Disord Tech 2003;16(1):38–43.
67. Goodman SM, Springer B, Guyatt G, et al. American College of Rheumatology/American Association of Hip and Knee Surgeons Guideline for the Perioperative Management of Antirheumatic Medication in Patients With Rheumatic Diseases Undergoing Elective Total Hip or Total Knee Arthroplasty. J Arthroplasty 2017;32(9):2628–38.
68. Joo P, Ge L, Mesfin A. Surgical management of the lumbar spine in rheumatoid arthritis. Glob Spine J 2020;10(6):767–74.
69. Imamudeen N, Basheer A, Iqbal AM, et al. Management of osteoporosis and spinal fractures: contemporary guidelines and evolving paradigms. Clin Med Res 2022;20(2):95–106.
70. Schousboe JT, Shepherd JA, Bilezikian JP, et al. Executive summary of the 2013 International Society for Clinical Densitometry Position Development Conference on bone densitometry. J Clin Densitom Oct-Dec 2013;16(4):455–66.
71. Sardar ZM, Coury JR, Cerpa M, et al. Best practice guidelines for assessment and management of osteoporosis in adult patients undergoing elective spinal reconstruction. Spine (Phila Pa 1976) 2022; 47(2):128–35.
72. Morris MT, Tarpada SP, Tabatabaie V, et al. Medical optimization of lumbar fusion in the osteoporotic patient. Arch Osteoporos 2018;13(1):26.
73. Dimar J, Bisson EF, Dhall S, et al. Congress of neurological surgeons systematic review and evidence-based guidelines for perioperative spine: preoperative osteoporosis assessment. Neurosurgery 2021;89(Suppl 1):S19–25.
74. Lee CK, Choi SK, An SB, et al. Influence of osteoporosis following spine surgery on Reoperation, Readmission, and Economic Costs: an 8-year Nationwide population-based study in Korea. World Neurosurg 2021;149:e360–8.
75. Guyot JP, Cizik A, Bransford R, et al. Risk factors for cardiac complications after spine surgery. Evid Based Spine Care J 2010;1(2):18–25.
76. Ahmad W, Fernandez L, Bell J, et al. Assessment of postoperative outcomes of spine fusion patients with history of cardiac disease. J Am Acad Orthop Surg 2022;30(8):e683–9.
77. Casper DS, Rihn JA. Preoperative risk stratification: who needs medical consultation? Spine (Phila Pa 1976) 2020;45(12):860–1.
78. Fleisher LA, Fleischmann KE, Auerbach AD, et al. ACC/AHA guideline on perioperative cardiovascular evaluation and management of patients undergoing noncardiac surgery: a report of the American College of Cardiology/American Heart Association Task Force on practice guidelines. J Am Coll Cardiol 2014;64(22):e77–137.

79. Nielsen PR, Jorgensen LD, Dahl B, et al. Prehabilitation and early rehabilitation after spinal surgery: randomized clinical trial. Clin Rehabil 2010;24(2):137–48.
80. Adogwa O, Elsamadicy AA, Sergesketter A, et al. The impact of chronic kidney disease on postoperative outcomes in patients undergoing lumbar decompression and fusion. World Neurosurg 2018;110:e266–70.
81. Friedman AL. Management of the surgical patient with end-stage renal disease. Hemodial Int 2003; 7(3):250–5.
82. Barrett N, Spencer S, McIvor J, et al. Subclavian stenosis: a major complication of subclavian dialysis catheters. Nephrol Dial Transpl 1988;3(4):423–5.
83. Hardy S, Lee SH, Terasaki PI. Sensitization. Clin Transpl 2001;271–8.
84. Galbusera M, Remuzzi G, Boccardo P. Treatment of bleeding in dialysis patients. Semin Dial 2009;22(3): 279–86.
85. Beyene RT, Derryberry SL Jr, Barbul A. The effect of comorbidities on wound healing. Surg Clin North Am 2020;100(4):695–705.

Printed and bound by CPI Group (UK) Ltd, Croydon, CR0 4YY

08/05/2025

01864715-0012